Molecular
Diagnosis
and Treatment
of Melanoma

Molecular Diagnosis and Treatment of Melanoma

edited by

John M. Kirkwood

University of Pittsburgh School of Medicine and
University of Pittsburgh Cancer Institute
Pittsburgh, Pennsylvania

MARCEL DEKKER, INC.   NEW YORK · BASEL · HONG KONG

Library of Congress Cataloging-in-Publication Data

Molecular diagnosis and treatment of melanoma / edited by John M. Kirkwood.
      p. cm.
      Includes bibliographical references and index.
      ISBN 0-8247-0102-X (alk. paper)
      1. Melanoma--Molecular diagnosis. I. Kirkwood, John M.
      [DLNM: 1. Melanoma--therapy. 2. Melanoma--diagnosis.
      3. Molecular Biology. QZ 200 M718331 1997]
      RC280.M37M65 1997
      616.99'477--dc21
      DNLM/DLC
      for Library of Congress   97-52827
                                                      CIP

This book is printed on acid-free paper.

Headquarters
Marcel Dekker, Inc.
270 Madison Avenue, New York, NY 10016
tel: 212-696-9000; fax: 212-685-4540

Eastern Hemisphere Distribution
Marcel Dekker AG
Hutgasse 4, Postfach 812, CH-4001 Basel, Switzerland
tel: 44-61-261-8482; fax: 44-61-261-8896

World Wide Web
http://www.dekker.com

The publisher offers discounts on this book when ordered in bulk quantities. For more information, write to Special Sales/Professional Marketing at the headquarters address above.

Current printing (last digit):
10 9 8 7 6 5 4 3 2 1

PRINTED IN THE UNITED STATES OF AMERICA

PREFACE

The field of melanoma research, like the proportions of the disease itself, is rapidly growing. Monographs dealing with melanoma have periodically been assembled, and over the years these have taken strongly epidemiological, pathological, surgical, or immunological perspectives. To date, however, few have approached basic and clinical investigations with a therapeutic multimodality perspective. This has been the rewarding challenge for the present volume, which is intended to bring together developments in areas that have currently achieved a meaningful therapeutic impact, or are soon anticipated to have major impact, upon the disease or its understanding at a basic level.

The contributors to this volume are leaders in their respective fields of investigation. They have each illuminated areas of controversy and added new insight to the basic molecular pathophysiology that bear on the diagnostic and therapeutic developments that will certainly continue to evolve in the next decade. Thus, the molecular investigation of melanoma progression is central to efforts that will someday yield molecular interventions capable of altering the onset of this disease. The study of early melanoma and the immune response it engenders in situ will illuminate both the molecular pathology underlying the disease and the immunological response that is inextricably entwined with the outcome of this pathology at the host level. The discussions of sentinel node mapping and selective lymph node dissection, as well as radiotherapy and radiosurgery, for this disease reveal the substantial changes in therapeutic paradigms for melanoma that have occurred over the past few years—since neither of these modalities had even been brought to systematic evaluation in melanoma until recently. The efforts to alter the course of the disease with chemotherapy and biologic therapy range from interferons to cytokines and now extend to vaccines able to induce consistent antibody response to defined gangliosides, and T-cell cytotoxic responses to protein and peptide antigens of melanoma. These agents have given clinical oncologists the tools to manipulate immune responses that are increasingly selective and to offer the prospect of improved cure and survival of this disease.

This volume is intended to introduce the major spheres of current melanoma investigation and to highlight the progress and issues that relate to melanoma biology, immunology, and therapeutics that presently occupy melanoma investigators worldwide. It is fitting that the volume begins and closes with considerations of the molecular biology and molecular pathology of the disease, including the primary and precursor atypical nevus, which will likely become a fruitful target of basic and therapeutic investigation research in the immediate future. We pay tribute to the earlier compilations in this field by Clark, Goldman, and Mastrangelo, Milton and McGovern, Ackerman, and Ferrone, but note that epidemiological, pathological and surgical, and basic immunological facets of the disease have been the focus of works of the 1960s, '70s, and '80s. Therapeutic discussions have risen to the masthead only recently, and the degree to which they may figure into future similar volumes will doubtless continue to increase as the work described in this volume bears results.

John M. Kirkwood

CONTENTS

Contents

CONTRIBUTORS

Michael B. Atkins, M.D. Director of the Biological Therapy and Melanoma Program, Division of Hematology/Oncology, Beth Israel Deaconess Medical Center and Harvard Medical School, Boston, Massachusetts

Dorothea Becker, Ph.D. Associate Professor, Department of Pathology, University of Pittsburgh, Pittsburgh, Pennsylvania

Jürgen C. Becker, M.D. Department of Dermatology, University of Würzburg, Würzburg, Germany

Agop Y. Bedikian, M.D. Internist and Associate Professor of Medicine, Department of Melanoma/Sarcoma Medical Oncology, The University of Texas M.D. Anderson Cancer Center, Houston, Texas

Andrea Brobeil, B.S. Cutaneous Oncology Program, Moffitt Cancer Center and Research Institute, University of South Florida, Tampa, Florida

Eva-Bettina Bröcker, M.D. Head, Department of Dermatology, University of Würzburg, Würzburg, Germany

David E. Elder, M.D. Department of Pathology, University of Pennsylvania Medical Center, Philadelphia, Pennsylvania

John C. Flickinger, M.D. Professor of Radiation Oncology and Neurological Surgery, University of Pittsburgh, Pittsburgh, Pennsylvania

Ulrich Keilholz, M.D. Department of Medicine V, University of Heidelberg, Heidelberg, Germany

John M. Kirkwood, M.D. Professor and Vice Chairman for Clinical Research, Department of Medicine, University of Pittsburgh School of Medicine; and Director, Melanoma Center, University of Pittsburgh Cancer Institute, Pittsburgh, Pennsylvania

Douglas Kondziolka, M.D., M.Sc., F.R.C.S.(C), F.A.C.S. Associate Professor, Department of Neurological Surgery and Radiation Oncology, University of Pittsburgh, Pittsburgh, Pennsylvania

Sewa Singh Legha, M.D., F.A.C.P. Professor of Medicine, Department of Melanoma/Sarcoma Medical Oncology, The University of Texas M.D. Anderson Cancer Center, Houston, Texas

Philip O. Livingston, M.D. Department of Medicine, Memorial Sloan-Kettering Cancer Center, New York, New York

Douglas S. Reintgen, M.D. Program Leader, Cutaneous Oncology, Moffitt Cancer Center and Research Institute, and Professor of Surgery, University of South Florida, Tampa, Florida

Ulrich Rodeck, M.D. The Wistar Institute, Philadelphia, Pennsylvania

John T. Seykora, M.D., Ph.D. Department of Pathology, University of Pennsylvania Medical Center, Philadelphia, Pennsylvania

Salvador Somaza, M.D. Visiting Assistant Professor, Department of Neurological Surgery, University of Pittsburgh, Pittsburgh, Pennsylvania

Walter J. Storkus, Ph.D. Associate Professor, Department of Surgery, University of Pittsburgh School of Medicine, Pittsburgh, Pennsylvania

Thomas Tüting, M.D. Department of Surgery, University of Pittsburgh School of Medicine, Pittsburgh, Pennsylvania

Martina Willhauck, Ph.D. Department of Medicine V, University of Heidelberg, Heidelberg, Germany

Molecular Diagnosis and Treatment of Melanoma

Part I
Molecular Features of the Biology of Melanoma

1

MOLECULAR FEATURES OF MELANOMA PROGRESSION

Ulrich Rodeck

The Wistar Institute
Philadelphia, Pennsylvania

Dorothea Becker

University of Pittsburgh
Pittsburgh, Pennsylvania

I. INTRODUCTION

Human melanoma is exemplary of malignant diseases that exhibit three important features: First, melanoma occurs sporadically in approximately 90% of cases and is the result of familial predisposition in about 10% of cases. Second, both the sporadic and familial forms of melanoma in more than 60% of all cases evolve in a stepwise fashion. And third, if melanoma is detected in its early stages, the patient is often cured by resection of the primary tumor.

During the past decade, two major research avenues have been pursued to gain an understanding of important molecular events that govern the onset and progression of this disease. First, genes have been identified whose expression is altered in malignant melanomas compared to normal melanocytes. Second, cytogenetic aberrations, detected in a large number of primary and metastatic melanomas of both familial and sporadic origin, have guided investigations to identify chromosomal loci harboring genes which are expressed in normal melanocytes but are deleted or inactivated in advanced-stage melanomas.

Genes known to be expressed in malignant melanomas control either the proliferation of the tumor cells or facilitate their interactions with the host environment. Thus, we will discuss molecular changes as they relate to (1) aberrant proliferation of melanoma cells, (2) tumorigenicity, invasion, and metastatic spread, and (3) host immune responses to melanoma cells. In particular, we will emphasize molecular features that are altered in melanocytic lesions in situ as opposed to those observed only in melanocytes and melanoma cells grown in vitro. This distinction is important because in vitro culturing conditions can significantly impair or alter the phenotype of these cells. Furthermore, we will outline potential therapeutic approaches aimed at interrupting molecular pathways of melanoma development.

In 1975, Clark and his colleagues (1) published the first

report which suggested that melanomas can develop in a stage-specific fashion. Based upon a combination of clinical and histopathologic criteria, the stages of melanocytic progression are defined as atypical (dysplastic) nevi; melanoma in the radial growth phase (RGP); melanoma in the vertical growth phase (VGP); and melanoma in the metastatic growth phase (MGP). RGP melanomas are characterized by superficial growth confined to the epidermal compartment. Thus, RGP melanomas do not metastasize and are therefore considered clinically benign tumors. In contrast, VGP melanomas represent malignant tumors as they invariably invade the dermis and often have the competence to metastasize. The ability to propagate normal melanocytes as well as cells derived from primary and metastatic melanomas in culture has greatly facilitated the characterization of molecular alterations specific to the different stages of melanoma progression.

II. GROWTH FACTORS/CYTOKINES AND THEIR RECEPTORS

In this section, we will discuss melanoma-derived growth-regulatory molecules associated with aberrant proliferation of advanced-stage melanomas. Specifically, these molecules represent genes which code for growth factors/cytokines, their receptors, and cell-cycle regulators.

When cultured in vitro, melanoma cells established from primary and metastatic melanoma specimens produce a variety of different growth factors/cytokines. The most prominent of these molecules are: basic fibroblast growth factor (bFGF); transforming growth factor alpha (TGF-α); transforming growth factor beta (TGF-β); platelet-derived growth factor A and B (PDGF-A and PDGF-B); and interleukins (IL) –1, –6, and –8 (2–6).

While melanoma cells produce these growth factors/cytokines constitutively, e.g., in the absence of exogenous peptides and/or hormones (3), growth factor/cytokine production by normal melanocytes grown in vitro depends upon exogenous stimulation provided by the addition of peptides/hormones to their culture medium. For example, TGF-β production by normal melanocytes requires the addition of fetal calf serum or defined growth factors such as insulin-like growth factor 1 (IGF-1), epidermal growth factor (EGF), and transferrin. Similarly, in vitro normal melanocytes synthesize very low levels of bFGF mRNA which do not suffice to sustain their proliferation. Thus, propagation of normal melanocytes in vitro requires the presence of exogenous bFGF in their culture medium (7).

The finding that melanoma cells but not normal melanocytes synthesize their own growth factors, and thus can proliferate in protein-free medium (7), suggests that, in situ, a switch from paracrine to autocrine growth-stimulatory mechanisms occurs concomitantly with melanocytic tumor progression. For example, all melanoma cell lines and specimens analyzed to date have been shown to express bFGF (3, 8; Becker et al, unpublished observation). To investigate the importance of this growth factor in the proliferation of melanomas, bFGF-specific neutralizing antibodies were injected into the cytoplasm of melanoma cells, which arrested their growth (8). Even more effective in inhibiting the proliferation of malignant melanomas were antisense oligodeoxynucleotides targeted against different regions of human bFGF mRNA (9).

Over the past several years, the study of growth requirements for malignant melanomas and normal melanocytes has also focused extensively upon the analysis of receptors to which growth factors/cytokines have to bind in order to initiate signal transduction and thus induce cell proliferation. For example, like the ligand bFGF, one of its receptors, fibroblast growth factor receptor 1 (FGFR-1) (10), is expressed at very low levels in normal melanocytes but at high levels in primary and metastatic melanomas (11). Furthermore, as in the case of bFGF, antisense oligonucleotide-induced inhibition of FGFR-1 expression arrested the proliferation of primary and metastatic melanomas and induced signs indicative of terminal differentiation (11). Recent investigations performed in vivo have demonstrated that antisense targeting of bFGF and FGFR-1 in malignant melanomas leads to the arrest and regression of tumor growth as a result of blocked melanoma angiogenesis and subsequent induction of necrosis (Wang and Becker; unpublished manuscript). Thus, attenuating melanoma angiogenesis may benefit patients with metastatic melanoma. In addition, inhibition of bFGF and FGFR-1, by themselves or in combination with known angiogenesis antagonists, may serve as adjuvant therapy for patients who have undergone resection for a primary melanoma and therefore are at an increased risk for tumor recurrence or, as is often the case, for developing metastases.

Like bFGF, TGF-β is another growth factor constitutively produced by melanoma cells (2,3). In situ, expression of the three isoforms of TGF-β (12) was detected in nevi and advanced-stage melanomas (13,14). However, while TGF-β1 was detected at comparable levels in nevi and malignant melanomas, expression of the isoforms of TGF-β2 and TGF-β3 appears to be up-regulated upon progression from RGP to VGP melanomas. Interestingly, TGF-β1 was found to inhibit the proliferation of most melanoma cells when added to their culture medium (15). This observation may suggest that, although this growth factor is produced by melanoma cells, its role is not to govern their own proliferation but to stimulate tumor angiogenesis and/or suppress immune responses as demonstrated in other biological systems. For example, in the case of glioblastomas, TGF-β2 was documented to inhibit the proliferation of T cells and autologous lymphokine activated killer (LAK) cells (16–18).

Another growth factor, expressed in approximately 50%

of melanoma cell lines, is PDGF-B (19). Like TGF-β, PDGF-B does not stimulate the growth of melanoma cells but rather acts on cells surrounding the tumor cells. For example, when overexpressed in a melanoma cell line by way of transfection, this growth factor did not stimulate cell proliferation (20). Yet, when these PDGF-B-transfected melanoma cells were injected into nude mice, the resulting tumors grew significantly larger than the controls. Upon histologic examination of the tumors, notable proliferation of fibroblasts and increased numbers of blood vessels were detected in the PDGF-B-transfected tumors but not in untransfected melanoma tumors. Furthermore, the increased blood vessel content was accompanied by significantly less intratumoral necrosis, underscoring the involvement of PDGF-B in the angiogenesis of these tumors.

Two other melanoma-derived growth factors that may also exert their mode of action in a paracrine fashion, are interleukin 6 (IL-6) (21) and melanoma-inhibitory-activity (MIA) (22). Both growth factors/cytokines are produced by melanoma cell lines, yet they inhibit the proliferation of melanoma cell lines when added to their culture medium (23,24). However, it has been suggested that increased levels of IL-6, detected in the sera of melanoma patients, may be linked to poor survival (25). Melanoma-inhibitory-activity was initially purified from conditioned media of several melanoma cell lines (26). The molecule does not reveal significant homology to other known growth factors/cytokines, and its role in melanoma development is as yet unknown.

Approximately 70% of cultured melanoma cell lines express the cytokine IL-10, whereas cultures of normal melanocytes produce such low levels of IL-10 mRNA that the cytokine itself cannot be detected in their media. Whether melanomas in situ synthesize IL-10, or whether it is produced by tumor-infiltrating lymphocytes, remains to be determined. IL-10 inhibits the expression of major histocompatibility (MHC) class I and II antigens on macrophages, followed by suppression of T-cell responses to specific antigens (26–30). Given this observation, it is possible that IL-10 may contribute to the suppression of melanoma-specific T-cell responses. In addition to IL-10, cultured melanoma cell lines express mRNAs for cytokines such as IL-1, IL-6, IL-8, granulocyte-macrophage-colony stimulating factor (GM-CSF), granulocyte-colony stimulating factor (G-CSF), and, in few cases, tumor necrosis factor-alpha (TNF-α) (4–6). However, with the exception of IL-8, it is not yet clear whether these cytokines are also produced by melanomas in situ.

Taken together, production of growth factors/cytokines exerting their functions in either an autocrine or a paracrine fashion is one of the prominent features associated with progression to advanced-stage melanomas. Thus, establishing strategies that will successfully interrupt these autonomous growth-regulatory pathways may provide an important basis for melanoma therapy and prevention.

III.   ONCOGENES AND TUMOR SUPPRESSOR GENES

Parallel to studies characterizing the role of growth factors/cytokines and their receptors in human melanomas, a major focus of molecular investigations has been the pursuit of nuclear and cytoplasmic oncogenes and their putative functions in early and advanced-stage melanomas. For example, early studies reported expression of activated oncogenes such as N-ras and H-ras in approximately 20% of metastatic melanomas (31–33). However, the fact that these structurally altered genes were detected only in the metastatic growth phase but not in any of the preceding stages of melanoma development makes it unlikely that these genes contribute to the onset of melanoma. Similar investigations which explored the role of proto-oncogenes such as a c-myc, c-myb, c-met, c-src and c-abl, failed to provide evidence of structural alterations in any of these genes in a substantial

TABLE 1

Expression of Genes in the Human Melanocytic System

	Melanocytes	Nevi	Melanomas	
			Primary	Metastatic
Growth Factors/Receptors				
bFGF	−	+	++	++
FGFR-1	+	+	++	++
TGF-β_1	+/−	+	+	+
TGF-β_2	−	+	++	++
TGF-β_3	−	+	++	++
PDGF-β				+/−
IL-1				+
IL-6			+	+
IL-8				+
IL-10				+
GM-CSF				+
TNF-α				+
MIA			+	+
Oncogenes				
N-ras	−	−	−	+
H-ras	−	−	−	+
Adhesion Molecules				
MUC-18	−	+	++	++
I-CAM	+	++	++	++
V-CAM		+	−	−
E-cadherin	+		−	−
N-cadherin	+	+	+	+
P-cadherin	+	+	+	+
$\alpha_v\beta_3$ integrin	−	−	+/−	+
Proteases				
tPA	−	−	+/−	++
uPA	−	−	+/−	++
Type IV Collagenase			+	++

number of primary and metastatic melanoma cell lines (34,35).

Over the past two decades, cytogenetic analyses of malignant melanomas, metastatic melanomas in particular, have provided evidence for recurring chromosomal changes involving, predominantly, chromosomes 1, 6, 7, 9, 10, and 11, in both familial and sporadic melanomas (36,37). The finding that these cytogenetic aberrations represent mostly deletions of the short arm of chromosome 1, the long arm of chromosome 6, and smaller deletions of the short and/or long arm of chromosomes 9, 10, and 11 prompted a search for genes that reside on these chromosomes and that, upon progression to advanced-stage melanomas, become inactivated or deleted.

Despite extensive efforts to identify putative tumor suppressors of melanomas that may reside on human chromosome 1p and/or 6q, such genes have not yet been isolated. On the other hand, a familial melanoma locus was mapped to chromosome 9p13-p22 (38,39), followed by the identification of a putative tumor-suppressor gene in 9p21 (40,41). This gene was found to be identical to the previously isolated CDK4/CDK6 cyclin-dependent kinase inhibitor, p16 (42). By binding to CDK4 and CDK6, p16 inhibits the ability of these kinases to interact with D cyclins and thereby inhibits passage through the G1 phase of the cell cycle (42). Thus, by functioning as a negative regulator of cell-cycle progression, homozygous deletions of, or mutations in, p16 render this gene a tumor suppressor as it becomes inactivated during malignant development. Between 60 and 70% of human melanoma cell lines were initially reported either to have lost both alleles of p16 or to contain point mutations in the gene (40,41). However, subsequent studies reported that these p16 aberrations were detected predominantly in cell lines but only at a low frequency in primary and metastatic melanoma specimens, suggesting that long-term culturing of established melanoma cell lines may select for cells with deleted or altered p16 (43). Furthermore, some isolates of normal human melanocytes, as well as benign compound nevi, which are not precursors of melanoma also demonstrated loss of this gene (44). Thus, while p16 mutations or deletions may contribute to the onset of familial melanomas, the role of this gene in sporadic melanomas is not yet fully understood. Other known tumor-suppressor genes such, as p53 and NF1, were found to be mutated or deleted in only a small number of melanoma cell lines (45–47) thus, ruling out the possibility that they contribute to or are causal to the development of melanoma.

Additional approaches to isolate candidate tumor suppressor genes focus on the application of subtractive cDNA hybridization and differential display to isolate as yet unknown genes that are expressed in normal melanocytes but not in malignant melanomas, and vice versa. These latter strategies were used recently to isolate several novel genes (48) which reside on human chromosomes 3p14, 19q13.1, and 2p14-p16 (49). The finding that these genes are expressed in normal human melanocytes but not in primary and metastatic melanomas (48,49) suggests that, upon progression to melanoma, they become down-regulated or inactivated. Although the function(s) of these genes is not yet known, their transfection into primary and metastatic melanoma cell lines may broaden our knowledge of events that lead to the onset and development of melanomas.

IV. ADHESION MOLECULES

The two major functions of adhesion molecules are to facilitate cell–cell contact and to attach cells to the extracellular matrix (ECM). In addition, adhesion molecules affect multiple cellular functions relevant to tumor development, such as cell migration, proliferation, differentiation, apoptosis (programmed cell death), and immune recognition (50). While cell adhesion molecules (CAMs) mediate cell–cell contact, integrins facilitate primarily ECM attachment.

Based upon their molecular features and functions, CAMs relevant to melanoma progression are composed of two categories of genes, namely the I-CAM, V-CAM, and N-CAM adhesion receptors, and the cadherins. Members of the C-CAM family of proteins, such as MUC18, I-CAM-1, and V-CAM, represent integral membrane glycoproteins encompassing extracellular, immunoglobulin-like (Ig) domain(s), followed by a transmembrane region and a short cytoplasmic tail. MUC18 is a 113 kd membrane glycoprotein whose expression in the melanocytic system becomes more frequent with increasing tumor thickness (51). While MUC18 expression is detected at comparable levels in dermal nevocytes of benign and atypical nevi (52), high-level expression of MUC18 in VGP melanomas has been reported to correlate with poor prognosis and the competence to metastasize (51). Similarly, I-CAM-1 expression was found to be upregulated in benign nevi (53) and in VGP and MGP melanomas when compared to normal melanocytes (53,54). In contrast, expression of V-CAM is downregulated as melanomas progress; as a result, it is not expressed in the majority of VGP melanomas (55).

Another family of adhesion molecules whose expression is altered concomitantly with progression to advanced-stage melanomas, are the homophilic cadherins. For example, normal melanocytes express E-cadherin, which mediates their adhesion to the surrounding keratinocytes (56). In contrast, in vitro and in vivo expression of E-cadherins in melanoma cells appears to be downregulated (56,57), raising the possibility that, concordant with melanocytic progression, loss of E-cadherin may help sever adhesion of the melanocytic cells from their surrounding keratinocytes. While E-cadherin is differentially expressed in melanocytes versus melanomas, N- and P-cadherins are expressed both in melanocytes and melanomas (57).

Among adhesion molecules that anchor melanocytic cells to the ECM, integrins have emerged as important players. They represent heterodimeric adhesion receptors, consisting of an α- and a β-subunit, both of which interact with molecules comprising the ECM such as laminin, fibronectin, and collagens (50). The finding that the β3-subunit of integrin is upregulated at the transition from RGP to VGP melanomas, both in vitro (58) and in vivo (59), has led to the suggestion that this molecule may serve as a progression marker of melanoma. In VGP and MGP melanomas, the β3-subunit of integrin is associated with the αv-subunit (60). Interestingly, some malignant melanoma cell lines which failed to express the αv-subunit of integrin were reported to be nontumorigenic in nude mice (61). However, not all melanomas require the expression of αvβ3 integrin to form tumors in nude mice (62) or to metastasize (60). Recent studies performed in vitro demonstrate that the expression of αvβ3 integrin is required for the survival of some melanoma cells in three-dimensional collagen matrices (63). These matrices provide a microenvironment that more closely resembles in vivo conditions than that of cell cultures grown in vitro on a plastic surface. Given these experimental conditions, melanoma cells which failed to express αvβ3 integrin underwent apoptosis, suggesting that, in vivo, αvβ3 integrin expression in advanced-stage melanomas may promote their survival by anchoring the cells to the ECM. In addition to αvβ3 integrin, integrins such as α4β1 and α5β1 are upregulated upon progression to advanced-stage melanomas, while α1β1, α2β1, and α6β4 are downregulated (59,64). Whether any of these integrins contribute to the progression of melanomas in situ remains to be elucidated.

V. PROTEASES

Deregulated expression of proteases by tumor cells has been associated with their capacity for local invasion and dissemination. In general, movement or invasion of tumor cells across the ECM barriers requires not only attachment of tumor cells to the ECM but also degradation and subsequent migration of the cells through the ECM. Melanoma cells have been documented to produce several proteolytic enzymes, including plasminogen activators and collagenases, which facilitate invasion.

Compared to melanoma cell lines established from VGP melanomas, metastatic melanoma cell lines express increased levels of tissue-type and urokinase-type plasminogen activators (tPA and uPA) (65–67). Similarly, in situ, expression of tPA and uPA is detected predominantly in advanced-stage melanomas (66,68,69). Evidence for a functional contribution of plasminogen activators in malignant melanomas was provided in studies performed with nude mice, which demonstrated that overexpression of the plasminogen activator inhibitor-2 in the injected melanoma cells prevented them from forming metastases (70).

Another proteolytic enzyme that is upregulated in metastatic melanoma cell lines is gelatinase/type IV collagenase (65), which has been suggested to be required for the growth of melanomas but not for their ability to form metastases (71).

VI.   CONCLUSION

Summarized in this review are the results of recent studies that have provided evidence for molecular alterations that occur concomitantly with progression from early melanocytic lesions to advanced-stage melanomas. In particular, these investigations have focused upon known genes, whose expression is altered in malignant melanomas compared to normal melanocytes. Some of these genes have emerged as important players in the proliferation and cell adhesion of primary and metastatic melanomas and, thus, may represent valuable targets for the intervention and prevention of melanomas. However, concordant with efforts to devise strategies to locally target these genes and thereby inhibit their expression in melanomas, it is important to identify additional, hitherto unknown genes which are involved in or causal to the onset and development of malignant melanomas.

REFERENCES

1. Clark WH, Ainsworth AM, Bernardino EA, Yang CH, Mihm MC, Reed RJ. The developmental biology of primary human malignant melanomas. Sem Oncol 1975; 2:83–103.
2. Albino AP, Davis BM, Nanus DM. Induction of growth factor RNA expression in human malignant melanoma: markers of transformation. Cancer Res 1991; 51:4815–4820.
3. Rodeck U, Melber K, Kath R, Menssen HD, Varello M, Atkinson B, Herlyn M. Constitutive expression of multiple growth factor genes by melanoma cells but not normal melanocytes. J Invest Dermatol 1991; 97:20–26.
4. Colombo MP, Maccalli C, Mattei S, Melani C, Radrizzani M, Parmiani G. Expression of cytokine genes, including IL-6, in human malignant melanoma cell lines. Melanoma Res 1992; 2:181–189.
5. Bennicelli JL, Guerry D. Production of multiple cytokines by cultured human melanomas. Exp Dermatol 1993; 2:186–190.
6. Mattei S, Colombo MP, Melani C, Silvani A, Parmiani G, Herlyn M. Expression of cytokine/growth factors and their receptors in human melanoma and melanocytes. Int J Cancer 1994; 56:853–857.
7. Halaban R, Ghosh S, Baird A. bFGF is the putative natural growth factor for human melanocytes. In Vitro Cell Dev Biol 1987; 23:47–52.
8. Halaban R, Kwon BS, Ghosh S, Delli BP, Baird A. bFGF as an autocrine growth factor for human melanomas. Oncogene Res 1988; 3:177–186.
9. Becker D, Meier CB, Herlyn M. Proliferation of human malignant melanomas is inhibited by antisense oligodeoxynu-

cleotides targeted against basic fibroblast growth factor. EMBO J 1989; 8:3685–3691.

10. Johnson DE, Lee PL, Lu J, Williams LT. Diverse forms of a receptor for acidic and basic fibroblast growth factors. Mol Cell Biol 1990; 10:4728–4736.

11. Becker D, Lee PL, Rodeck U, Herlyn M. Inhibition of the fibroblast growth factor receptor 1 (FGFR-1) gene in human melanocytes and malignant melanomas leads to inhibition of proliferation and signs indicative of differentiation. Oncogene 1992; 7:2303–2313.

12. Massague J. The transforming growth factor-β family. Ann Rev Cell Biol 1990; 6:597–641.

13. Reed JA, McNutt NS, Prieto VG, Albino AP. Expression of transforming growth factor-β 2 in malignant melanoma correlates with the depth of tumor invasion. Implications for tumor progression. Am J Pathol 1994; 145:97–104.

14. Van Belle P, Rodeck U, Nuamah I, Halpern AC, Elder DE. Melanoma-associated expression of TGF-β isoforms. Am J Pathol 1996; 148:1887–1894.

15. Rodeck U, Bossler A, Graeven U, Fox F, Nowell P, Kari C. Transforming growth factor-β production and responsiveness in normal human melanocytes and melanoma cells. Cancer Res 1994; 54:575–581.

16. De Martin R, Haendler B, Hofer WR, Gaugitsch H, Wrann M, Schlusener H, Seifert JM, Bodmer S, Fontana A, Hofer E. Complementary DNA for human glioblastoma-derived T cell suppressor factor, a novel member of the transforming growth factor-β gene family. EMBO J 1987; 6:3673–3677.

17. Wrann M, Bodmer S, de Martin R, Siepl C, Hofer WR, Frei K, Hofer E, Fontana A. T cell suppressor factor from human glioblastoma cells is a 12.5-kd protein closely related to transforming growth factor-β. EMBO J 1987; 6:1633–1636.

18. Ruffini PA, Rivoltini L, Silvani A, Boiardi A, Parmiani G. Factors, including transforming growth factor β, released in the glioblastoma residual cavity, impair activity of adherent lymphokine-activated killer cells. Cancer Immunol Immunotherapy 1993; 36:409–416.

19. Westermark B, Johnsson A, Paulsson Y, Betsholtz C, Heldin C-H, Herlyn M, Rodeck U, Koprowski H. Human melanoma

cells of primary and metastatic origin express the genes encoding the constituent chains of PDGF and produce a PDGF-like growth factor. Proc Natl Acad Sci USA 1986; 83: 7197–7200.

20. Forsberg K, Valyi-Nagy I, Heldin CH, Herlyn M, Westermark B. Platelet-derived growth factor (PDGF) in oncogenesis: development of a vascular connective tissue stroma in xeno-transplanted human melanoma producing PDGF-BB. Proc Natl Acad Sci USA 1993; 90:393–397.

21. Armstrong CA, Murray N, Kennedy M, Koppula SV, Tara D, Ansel JC. Melanoma-derived interleukin 6 inhibits in vivo melanoma growth. J Invest Dermatol 1994; 102:278–284.

22. Blesch A, Bosserhoff AK, Apfel R, Behl C, Hessdoerfer B, Schmitt A, Jachimczak P, Lottspeich F, Buettner R, Bogdahn U. Cloning of a novel malignant melanoma-derived growth-regulatory protein, MIA. Cancer Res 1994; 54:5695–5701.

23. Lu C, Vickers MF, Kerbel RS. Interleukin 6: a fibroblast-derived growth inhibitor of human melanoma cells from early but not advanced stages of tumor progression. Proc Natl Acad Sci USA 1992; 89:9215–9219.

24. Lu C, Kerbel RS. Interleukin-6 undergoes transition from paracrine growth inhibitor to autocrine stimulator during human melanoma progression. J Cell Biol 1993; 120:1281–1288.

25. Tartour E, Dorval T, Mosseri V, Deneux L, Mathiot C, Brailly H, Montero F, Joyeux I, Pouillart P, Fridman WH. Serum interleukin 6 and C-reactive protein levels correlate with resistance to IL-2 therapy and poor survival in melanoma patients. Br J Cancer 1994; 69:911–913.

26. de Waal Malefyt R, Haanen J, Spits H, Roncarolo MG, te Velde A, Figdor C, Johnson K, Kastelein R, Yssel H, de Vries JE. Interleukin 10 (IL-10) and viral IL-10 strongly reduce antigen-specific human T cell proliferation by diminishing the antigen-presenting capacity of monocytes via downregulation of class II major histocompatibility complex expression. J Exp Med 1991; 174:915–924.

27. de Waal Malefyt R, Abrams J, Bennett B, Figdor CG, de Vries JE. Interleukin 10 (IL-10) inhibits cytokine synthesis by human monocytes: an autoregulatory role of IL-10 produced by monocytes. J Exp Med 1991; 174:1209–1220.

28. Bogdan C, Vodovotz Y, Nathan C. Macrophage deactivation by interleukin 10. J Exp Med 1991; 174:1549–1555.
29. de Waal Malefyt R, Yssel H, de Vries JE. Direct effects of IL-10 on subsets of human CD4+ T cell clones and resting T cells. Specific inhibition of IL-2 production and proliferation. J Immunol 1993; 150:4754–4765.
30. Matsuda M, Salazar F, Petersson M, Masucci G, Hansson J, Pisa P, Zhang QJ, Masucci MG, Kiessling R. Interleukin 10 pretreatment protects target cells from tumor- and allo-specific cytotoxic T cells and downregulates HLA class I expression. J Exp Med 1994; 180:2371–2376.
31. Albino AP, Nanus DM, Davis ML, McNutt NS. Lack of evidence of Ki-ras codon 12 mutations in melanocytic lesions. J Cutan Pathol 1991; 18:273–278.
32. Dicker AP, Volkenandt M, Albino AP. Mutational analysis of human NRAS genes in malignant melanoma: rapid methods for oligonucleotide hybridization and manual and automated direct sequencing of products generated by the polymerase chain reaction. Genes. Chromosomes Cancer 1990; 1: 257–269.
33. Albino AP, Nanus DM, Mentle IR, Cordon CC, McNutt NS, Bressler J, Andreeff M. Analysis of ras oncogenes in malignant melanoma and precursor lesions: correlation of point mutations with differentiation phenotype. Oncogene 1989; 4: 1363–1374.
34. Linnenbach AJ, Huebner K, Reddy EP, Herlyn M, Parmiter AH, Nowell PC, Koprowski H. Structural alteration in the MYB proto-oncogene and deletion within the gene encoding alpha-type protein kinase C in human melanoma cell lines. Proc Natl Acad Sci USA 1988; 85:74–78.
35. Husain Z, Fitz GG, Wick MM. Comparison of cellular proto-oncogene activation and transformation-related activity of human melanocytes and metastatic melanoma. J Invest Dermatol 1990; 95:571–575.
36. Parmiter AH, Nowell PC. The cytogenetics of human malignant melanoma and premalignant lesions. Cancer Treat Res 1988; 43:47–61.
37. Trent JM. Cytogenetics of human malignant melanoma. Cancer Metast Rev 1991; 10:103–113.

38. Fountain JW, Karayiorgou M, Ernstoff MS, Kirkwood JM, Vlock DR, Titus-Ernstoff L, Bouchard B, Vijayasaradhi S, Houghton AN, Lahti J, Kidd VJ, Housman DE. Homozygous deletions within human chromosome band 9p21 in melanoma. Proc Natl Acad Sci USA 1992; 89:10557–10561.

39. Cannon-Albright LA, Goldgar DE, Meyer LJ, Lewis CM, Anderson DE, Fountain JW, Hegi ME, Wiseman RW, Petty EM, Bale AE, Olopade OI, Diaz MO, Kwiatkowski DJ, Piepkorn MW, Zone JJ, Skolnick MH. Assignment of a locus for familial melanoma, MLM, to chromosome 9p13-p22. Science 1992; 258:1148–1152.

40. Kamb A, Shattuck-Eidens D, Eeles R, Liu Q, Gruis NA, Ding W, Hussey C, Tran T, Miki Y, Weaver-Feldhaus J, McClure M, Aitken JF, Anderson DE, Bergman W, Frants R, Goldgar DE, Green A, MacLennan R, Martin NG, Meyer LJ, Youl P, Zone JJ, Skolnick MH, Cannon-Albright LA. Analysis of the p16 gene (CDKN2) as a candidate for the chromosome 9p melanoma susceptibility locus. Nature Genet 1994; 8:22–26.

41. Nobori T, Miura K, Wu DJ, Lois A, Takabayashi K, Carson DA. Deletions of the cyclin-dependent kinase-4 inhibitor gene in multiple human cancers. Nature 1994; 368:753–756.

42. Serrano M, Hannon GJ, Beach D. A new regulatory motif in cell-cycle control causing specific inhibition of cyclin D/CDK4. Nature 1993; 366:704–707.

43. Ohta M, Nagai H, Shimizu M, Rasio D, Berd D, Mastrangelo M, Singh AD, Shields JA, Shields CL, Croce CM, Huebner K. Rarity of somatic and germline mutations of the cyclin-dependent kinase 4 inhibitor gene, CDK4l, in melanoma. Cancer Res 1994; 54:5269–5272.

44. Wang Y, Becker D. Differential expression of the cyclin-dependent kinase inhibitors p16 and p21 in the human melanocytic system. Oncogene 1996; 12:1069–1075.

45. Volkenandt M, Schlegel U, Nanus DM, Albino AP. Mutational analysis of the human p53 gene in malignant melanoma. Pigment Cell Res 1991; 4:35–40.

46. Andersen LB, Fountain JW, Gutmann DH, Tarle SA, Glover TW, Dracopoli NC, Housman DE, Collins FS. Mutations in the neurofibromatosis 1 gene in sporadic malignant melanoma cell lines. Nature Genet 1993; 3:118–121.

47. Albino AP, Vidal MJ, McNutt NS, Shea CR, Prieto VG, Nanus DM, Palmer JM, Hayward NK. Mutation and expression of the p53 gene in human malignant melanoma. Melanoma Res 1994; 4:35–45.
48. Gratas C, Herlyn M, Becker D. Isolation and analysis of novel human melanocyte-specific cDNA clones. DNA and Cell Biol 1994; 13:515–519.
49. Gratas C, Li X, Wang Y, Francke U, Becker D. Chromosomal assignment of three human melanocyte-specific genes. Int J Oncol 1996; 9:481–485.
50. Albelda SM, Buck CA. Integrins and other cell adhesion molecules. Faseb J 1990; 4:2868–2880.
51. Lehmann JM, Riethmuller G, Johnson JP. MUC18, a marker of tumor progression in human melanoma, shows sequence similarity to the neural cell adhesion molecules of the immunoglobulin superfamily. Proc Natl Acad Sci USA 1989; 86: 9891–9895.
52. Wang Y, Rao U, Mascari R, Richards TJ, Panson AJ, Edington HD, Shipe-Spotloe JM, Donnelly SS, Kirkwood JM, Becker D. Molecular analysis of melanoma precursor lesions. Cell Growth & Differentation. In press.
53. Denton KJ, Stretch JR, Gatter KC, Harris AL. A study of adhesion molecules as markers of progression in malignant melanoma. J Pathol 1992; 167:187–191.
54. Kageshita T, Yoshii A, Kimura T, Kuriya N, Ono T, Tsujisaki M, Imai K, Ferrone S. Clinical relevance of I-CAM-1 expression in primary lesions and serum of patients with malignant melanoma. Cancer Res 1993; 53:4927–4932.
55. van Duinen CM, van den Broek LJ, Vermeer BJ, Fleuren GJ, Bruijn JA. The distribution of cellular adhesion molecules in pigmented skin lesions. Cancer 1994; 73:2131–2139.
56. Tang A, Eller MS, Hara M, Yaar M, Hirohashi S, Gilchrest BA. E-cadherin is the major mediator of human melanocyte adhesion to keratinocytes in vitro. J Cell Sci 1994; 107:983–992.
57. Hsu M-Y, Wheelock MJ, Johnson KR, Herlyn M. Shifts in cadherin profiles in normal human melanocytes and melanomas. J Invest Dermatol, Symp Proc 1996; vol. 1, 188–194.
58. Albelda SM, Mette SA, Elder DE, Stewart R, Damjanovich L, Herlyn M, Buck CA. Integrin distribution in malignant

melanoma: association of the β 3 subunit with tumor progression. Cancer Res 1990; 50:6757–6764.

59. Danen EH, Ten Berge PJ, Van Muijen GN, Van't Hof-Grootenboer AE, Brocker EB, Ruiter DJ. Emergence of α5β1 fibronectin- and αυβ3 vitronectin-receptor expression in melanocytic tumour progression. Histopathology 1994; 24: 249–256.

60. Danen EH, Jansen KF, Van Kraats AA, Cornelissen IM, Ruiter DJ, Van Muijen GN. Alpha v-integrins in human melanoma: gain of αυβ3 and loss of αυβ5 are related to tumor progression in situ but not to metastatic capacity of cell lines in nude mice. Int J Cancer 1995; 61:491–496.

61. Felding-Habermann B, Mueller BM, Romerdahl CA, Cheresh DA. Involvement of integrin αυ gene expression in human melanoma tumorigenicity. J Clin Invest 1992; 89:2018–2022.

62. Boukerche H, Benchaibi M, Berthier-Vergnes O, Lizard G, Bailly M, Bailly M, McGregor JL. Two human melanoma cell-line variants with enhanced in vivo tumor growth and metastatic capacity do not express the β3 integrin subunit. Eur J Biochem 1994; 220:485–491.

63. Montgomery AM, Reisfeld RA, Cheresh DA. Integrin αυβ3 rescues melanoma cells from apoptosis in three-dimensional dermal collagen. Proc Natl Acad Sci USA 1994; 91:8856–8860.

64. Schadendorf D, Gawlik C, Haney U, Ostmeier H, Suter L, Czarnetzki BM. Tumour progression and metastatic behaviour in vivo correlates with integrin expression on melanocytic tumours. J Pathol 1993; 170:429–434.

65. Herlyn D, Iliopoulos D, Jensen PJ, Parmiter A, Baird J, Hotta H, Adachi K, Ross AH, Jambrosic J, Koprowski H, et al. In vitro properties of human melanoma cells metastatic in nude mice. Cancer Res 1990; 50:2296–2302.

66. van Muijen GN, Danen EH, de Vries TJ, Quax PH, Verheijen JH, Ruiter DJ. Properties of metastasizing and nonmetastasizing human melanoma cells. Cancer Res 1995; 139: 105–122.

67. Colombi M, Bellotti D, De Petro G, Barlati S. Plasminogen activators in nude mice xenotransplanted with human tumorigenic cells. Inv Metast 1995; 15:22–33.

68. Delbaldo C, Masouye I, Saurat JH, Vassalli JD, Sappino AP.

Plasminogen activation in melanocytic neoplasia. Cancer Res 1994; 54:4547–4552.

69. de Vries TJ, Quax PH, Denijn M, Verrijp KN, Verheijen JH, Verspaget HW, Weidle UH, Ruiter DJ, van Muijen GN. Plasminogen activators, their inhibitors, and urokinase receptor emerge in late stages of melanocytic tumor progression. Am J Pathol 1994; 144:70–81.

70. Mueller BM, Yu YB, Laug WE. Overexpression of plasminogen activator inhibitor 2 in human melanoma cells inhibits spontaneous metastasis in scid/scid mice. Proc Natl Acad Sci USA 1995; 92:205–209.

71. Montgomery AM, Mueller BM, Reisfeld RA, Taylor SM, De Clerck YA. Effect of tissue inhibitor of the matrix metalloproteinases-2 expression on the growth and spontaneous metastasis of a human melanoma cell line. Cancer Res 1994; 54: 5467–5473.

2

IMMUNOLOGIC FEATURES OF PROGRESSION IN MELANOMA

Jürgen C. Becker and Eva-Bettina Bröcker

University of Würzburg
Würzburg, Germany

I. INTRODUCTION

Consensus holds that melanoma cells are antigenic, since they express tumor-associated antigens which are recognized by syngeneic T cells (1–4). Furthermore, cellular components that should be able to reject the tumor, i.e., T lymphocytes and macrophages, infiltrate both primary and metastatic tumors (5,6). Nevertheless, the prognosis for melanoma, if it is not cured by surgical resection, is one of the most unfavorable in medicine (7). The coexistence of tumor-specific immunity with a progressing tumor remains a major paradox of tumor immunology. This enigma is most evident in partially regressing melanoma, where efficient eradication of tumor cells occurs in close vicinity to uncontrolled tumor growth (8,9). In order to delineate the mechanisms used by melanoma cells to escape the host immune surveillance, we first describe the events involved in induction and maintenance of an antitumor T-cell response. In the second part of this chapter, a number of such immune escape mechanisms are discussed.

II. T-CELL MEDIATED IMMUNE RESPONSES

A. Antigen Presentation

A successful antitumor T-cell response involves induction, recruitment, and effector function of T cells. The action of T cells is dependent upon their ability to recognize neoplastic cells. Such neoplastic cells are identified by the expression of specific peptides on the cell surface in association with two distinct classes of major histocompatibility complex (MHC) molecules. The MHC class I pathway is operative in almost all cells and allows the immune system to monitor tissues for the presence of viral infections and tumors and subsequently activate cytotoxic T lymphocytes (CTLs) to kill such cells (10). In this process, proteins are hydrolyzed in the cytosol by a large multicatalytic proteolytic complex of 28 subunits, called the proteasome, resulting in oligopeptides which are transferred into the endoplasmatic reticulum by the transporter associated with antigen processing (TAP) (11,12). Newly synthesized MHC class I heavy chains assemble in the endoplasmatic reticulum with β2-microglobulin and a membrane-bound protein, calnexin (13). In this complex, the MHC class I molecule is retained within the endoplasmatic reticulum. Release of the MHC class I molecule from calnexin is dependent on the binding of a peptide, thereby completing the folding of the MHC class I molecule. The peptide/MHC complex is then transported through the Golgi complex to the cell surface.

The general view has been that the MHC class I pathway is exclusively concerned with monitoring endogenously synthesized proteins of a cell, whereas the class II pathway presents exogenous antigens (14). This segregation is important to prevent CTLs from killing healthy cells that have been exposed to foreign antigens. However, although somatic cells can efficiently stimulate effector CTLs, they are poor antigen-presenting cells for naive T cells since they lack costimulatory molecules, e.g., B7-1 and B7-2 (CD80 and CD86), as well as adhesion receptors (15,16). Finally, somatic cells do not migrate into lymphoid tissues, where immune responses are thought to be initiated (17). This point is particularly important since naive cells, as opposed to memory or activated T cells, do not access peripheral tissue (18). Thus, in the case of a malignant somatic cell, the question of how CTL responses are initiated remains. A number of recent reports implicate phagocytes, e.g., macrophages or dentritic cells, with the priming of CTL responses against malignant cells (19). Antigens in association with cell debris derived from malignant cells are internalized into such cells by phagocytosis or macropinocytosis, depending on the size and solubility of the particle (20). The antigen is then transferred from phagosomes into the cytosol and becomes available to the classical MHC class I presentation pathway described above. Tumor-derived antigens can thus be presented to naive T cells by a "professional" antigen-presenting cell (APC) initiating an effective CTL response.

As mentioned above, MHC class II molecules primarily present exogenous peptides to CD4+ T cells. Newly synthesized MHC class II α and β chains form heterodimers in the absence of peptide and associate with a third component, the invariant chain, in the endoplasmatic reticulum; this complex is transported through the Golgi stacks to endosomes. The invariant chain prevents the binding of endogenous peptides to MHC class II molecules until it is cleaved by proteases in an endosomal post-Golgi compartment, allowing peptide-class II complexes to be formed and transported to the cell surface (21). These peptides arise from limited proteolytic degradation of exogenous antigens by enzymes such as Cathepsin D and B. However, the mechanism by which these antigen fragments are loaded onto MHC class II molecules is not fully understood but appears to involve chaperone proteins (22).

B. The T-Cell Receptor/CD3 Complex

The MHC/peptide complex is recognized by the T-cell receptor (TCR); this process leads to activation of mature T cells. Each T cell bears about 30,000 TCR molecules on its surface. The TCR consists of 2 different polypeptide chains, termed the TCR α and β chains, bound to one another by a disulfide bond in a structure that is highly homologous to a F_{ab} fragment of an immunoglobulin (Ig) (23). The TCR α- and β-chain genes are composed of discrete segments, i.e., variable (V), diversity (D), joining (J), and constant (C) segments, which are joined by somatic recombination during development of the T cell (24,25). For the α-chain, like Ig light chains, a V_α gene segment rearranges to a J_α gene segment to create a functional exon. Transcription and splicing of the VJ_α exon to $C\alpha$ generates the mRNA that is translated to yield the α-chain. For β chains, similar to the Ig heavy chain, the variable domain is encoded in three gene segments V_β, D_β, and J_β. Rearrangement of these gene segments generates a functional exon that is transcribed and then spliced to join $VDJ\beta$ to $C\beta$. Comparing the origins of diversity in the TCR with those in Ig demonstrates that most of the variability in TCRs occurs within the junctional regions encoded by D, J, and N nucleotides. This region encodes the complementary determining region (CDR) 3 loop in Ig that forms the center of the antigen binding site (26). Thus, when superimposing the proposed structure of the TCR on its ligand—i.e., the MHC/peptide complex—the most variable region of the receptor lies over the most variable part of the ligand, the bound peptide.

Neither chain of the TCR has a large cytoplasmic domain that might serve to signal the cell that it has bound antigen. Instead, this function is carried out by a complex of proteins, named CD3, that are stably associated with the TCR. The CD3 complex consists of six invariant chains: CD3γ, CD3δ, two copies of CD3ε, and a CD3ζ homodimer (23). In about 20% of chains, the ζ homodimer may be substituted by a ζ/η heterodimer (27). No recognizable enzymatic domain has been identified in any of these chains, but they contain the antigen-recognition activation motif (ARAM) or the tyrosine-based activation motif (TAM) that has been demonstrated to have signaling function (28). Following phosphorylation by protein tyrosine kinases (PTK), ARAMs interact with the antigen receptor and thereby recruit to it the Syk family tyrosine kinases p72^{syk} and ζ-associated protein-70 (ZAP-70) (29,30). These kinases are distinguished from the Src family kinases by the absence of a myristylation signal and the negative regulatory carboxy-terminal tyrosine, as well as by the presence of a second SH2 domain (30).

C. Co-Receptors

During antigen recognition, CD4 and CD8 molecules associate on the cell surface with components of the TCR and function as co-receptors (28). The single-chair CD4 molecules bind to an invariant domain of MHC class II molecules; such binding leads to activation of the CD4-associated Src family kinase p56^{lck} (31). The CD8 molecule consists of two different chains, binds to MHC class I, and is also associated with p56[lck] at its cytoplasmatic tail (32). When T cells recognize the specific peptide/MHC complex, the TCR/CD3 complex aggregates with either CD4 or CD8. The cytoplasmatic tails of these molecules are brought together in this process, leading to triggering of the T cell. It requires about 100 specific peptide/MHC complexes to trigger a mature T cell that expresses suitable coreceptors; if these are not present, about 10,000 identical peptide/MHC complexes would be required which means approximately 10% of all the MHC molecules on the cell surface (33).

D. T-Cell Activation

TCR ligation by peptide/MHC complexes leads to aggregation of TCR complex with the CD4 or CD8 coreceptors, which is followed by phosphorylation of ARAMs within CD3ζ by p56[lck] (28,31,32). CD3ζ then binds and activates the Syk-family kinase ZAP-70 (29,30). Activated ZAP-70 phosphorylates the adapter molecule p36, which binds to phospholipase Cγ1, thus regulating inositol phospholipid metabolism and protein kinase C signaling pathways. p36 also binds the Src homology (SH) 2 domain of the adapter protein Grb2. The SH3 domain of Grb2 binds a guanine exchange protein for p21[ras], Sos (28,32,34). Thereby, p36-Grb2-Sos links TCR-mediated signaling to the p21[ras]/Raf-1/ERK kinase cascade. The nuclear targets for each signaling pathway are transcriptional activator proteins, i.e., AP-1, NF-kB or NF-ATp. Cytokine genes such as interleukin 2 require the coordinate action of multiple transcriptional factors for activation (35–37).

In naïve T cells, preceding cytokine production and proliferation, signals generated through the TCR are not sufficient for full activation (15,38). Additional antigen-nonspecific costimulatory signals are required. Interactions between CD28 on the T cell and CD80 or CD86 on the APC appear to provide the major costimulatory signals. Early events in CD28-mediated signals transduction may include binding and activation of phosphoinositide 3-kinase and the mitogen-activated protein kinase (MAPK) JNK1 (38). The latter protein kinase phosphorylates the transcription factor c-Jun and thereby activates AP-1 and NF-ATp. Furthermore, CD28 stimulation leads to the induction of an activating transcription factor, the CD28 responsive complex, which binds to the IL-2 promoter (39). TCR- and CD28-mediated signals seem to be integrated at the level of induction of cytokine gene transcription.

III. T-CELL MEDIATED IMMUNE RESPONSES TO MELANOMA

A. Tumor-Infiltrating Lymphocytes

Melanomas are often characterized by lymphocyte infiltration which has been reported to be associated with a good prognosis (5,6). A number of investigators employing T-cell cloning technology were able to isolate autologous melanoma-specific CTL clones from patients with melanoma (1,3). These clones conform with all the tenets of T-cell-mediated recognition of antigen—e.g., selectively recognizing a putative antigen in association with the self-MHC molecule. Some of these CTL clones were also found to recognize certain allogeneic melanoma cells (40). These cell lines, however, shared a MHC class I molecule between them; in most cases this MHC-restriction element was HLA-A2, a haplotype that is expressed in approximately 50% of the Caucasian population.

Studies of the TCR repertoire expressed by tumor-infiltrating lymphocytes (TIL) were initiated to analyze whether melanoma cells may elicit, as result of antigenic stimulation, an in situ immune response. Such a response should be dominated by oligoclonal T cells thus, exhibiting only a limited set of TCR β chains (41). For this purpose, a semiquantitative polymerase chain reaction (PCR) approach was adopted to identify tumor-reactive intratumoral T-cell populations, either locally recruited or undergoing clonal expansion from nonspecific lymphocytic infiltrates that are contributing to a polyclonal background. In most studies, frequencies obtained from TCRV or TCRβV subfamilies in TIL were compared with those in peripheral blood lymphocytes or normal tissues of the same patients. These studies revealed that, in general, 1 to 3 TCRV or TCRβV regions are over-represented in TIL and that the patterns differ in each patient (41–44). Since this observation can easily be explained by differences of MHC haplotypes, studies were initiated in which melanoma patients were matched for HLA-A2 expression (45). It was found that TCRβV14 was overexpressed in all lesions studied; TCRβV14 was not overexpressed in HLA-A2 negative patients. Subsequent analysis suggested that recognition of the shared melanocytic differentiation antigens MART-1/Melan-A or gp100 could be mediated by TCRβV14-expressing T cells (46). Characterization of TCR rearrangements of TIL obtained from primary tumors or subsequent metastases revealed that TCRV or TCRβV subfamilies that were highly expressed in primary tumors were not overexpressed in metastases (47). Recently, we were able to demonstrate that these differences might actually be present in the primary tumor but become apparent only when different parts of the tumor are analyzed separately (48). Subcloning and sequencing of the CDR3 of the overexpressed TIL TCRβV subfamilies demonstrated that these are indeed due to clonal expansion of these T cells. In contrast, the corresponding TCRβV transcripts of peripheral blood lymphocytes were polyclonal, and no sequences identical to the dominant one expressed in TIL could be detected (41).

B. Tumor-Associated Antigens

The overexpression of distinct TCRV or TCRβV subfamilies as revealed by direct assessment of the TCR repertoire reflects the recognition of tumor-specific antigens by clonal-expanded T cells. One of the barriers to identifying molecules in tumor cells recognized by T cells is the inability to use the TCR directly as an affinity reagent. Thierry Boon et al. developed a method to overcome this limitation by cloning the genes encoding antigens recognized by tumor-specific CTL clones (49). This technique is based on two crucial processes. The first is to transfect a complementary DNA library derived from the tumor into either antigen loss variants of the same tumor or Cos cells together with genes encoding the appropriate MHC class I. The second was to identify the antigen in CTL stimulation assays. To date, three different types of tumor antigens have been identified from melanoma patients using this method (2). They can be classified as shared tissue-specific differentiation antigens, nonmutated tumor-specific antigens, or mutated tumor-specific antigens. The most common responses appear to be directed not at tumor specific antigens, but rather at differentiation antigens that are specific to normal melanocytes and melanomas. These include tyrosinase, MART-1/Melan-A, gp100, and gp75 (46,50–52). The second category of tumor antigens seem to be more specific for neoplastic cells in that they are expressed in a large proportion of melanomas but are not expressed in other adult, normal tissues (with the exception of the testes). This category of antigens include the MAGE, BAGE, and GAGE gene families (53–55). Why the genes encoding these antigens are turned on in melanoma cells is not fully understood but might be due to a dysregulated state of gene expression inherent to tumors in general, since these antigens are found in a wide range of neoplasms beyond melanoma. In the case of MAGE, it has been demonstrated that demethylation of the binding site for the transcriptional activator protein Ets within the MAGE-promoter leads to gene transcription. Among the antigens which are derived from mutated genes, an interesting example is a peptide derived from a mutated CDK4 gene (56). It has been demonstrated that the mutation is in a region to which the tumor-suppressor antigen product p16 is binding; thus, the mutated CDK4 in this patient was incapable of binding p16.

These observations raise the question of why potentially reactive CTLs fail to exert sufficient cytotoxicity against antigenic melanoma cells to prevent tumor progression in vivo. A number of mechanisms may be operational in the immune escape of melanoma. These will be examined, based on our present knowledge of T-cell-mediated antitumor responses.

IV. MECHANISMS OF TUMOR ESCAPE FROM IMMUNE RECOGNITION

A. MHC Class I

As discussed above, MHC class I antigens are essential for immune recognition of malignant cells. Structural or functional abnormalities of these molecules may have a negative impact on T-cell recognition and control of tumor growth. In the course of local and systemic progression of melanoma, an increasing proportion of tumor cells lack detectable MHC class I (HLA-A, B, C) molecules on the cell surface (57,58). This was demonstrated in vivo by immunohistological studies employing monoclonal antibodies against epitopes on the constant invariant part of this molecule; 16% of primary and 58% of metastatic melanoma lesions failed to be stained by these antibodies (59,60). The higher incidence of loss of class I antigens in metastatic compared with primary lesion is not unique to melanoma; this also has been observed in other neoplasms (58).

The loss of MHC class I expression may be caused by lack of β_2-microglobulin synthesis or by the synthesis of a truncated form of this protein unable to associate with class I heavy chains. Such defects have been shown for a number of melanoma cell lines (61,62). For example, the lack of HLA class I expression by a subline of SK-MEL-33 is caused by a unique lesion in the β_2-microglobulin gene (62). Sequencing of this mutated β_2-microglobulin mRNA detected a guanosine deletion on position 323 in codon 76 that causes a frameshift with a subsequent introduction of a stop codon at a position-54 base upstream of the normal position of the stop codon. The loss of 18 amino acids and the change of 6 amino acids are likely to cause marked changes in the structure of the polypeptide, which may account for the inability of β_2-microglobulin to associate with MHC class I heavy chains. A similar defect had been shown for another melanoma cell line, FO-1, which showed a gross deletion of the 5' region and a portion of the coding region of the β_2-microglobulin gene molecules, preventing its transcription and, consequently, the expression of MHC class I (61). Deletions in the putative promoter region upstream of the TATA box of the β_2-microglobulin gene in melanoma cells are the further basis for reduced transcription (58). The role of β_2-microglobulin in the lack of class I expression has been shown conclusively by restoration of class I expression following transfection of melanoma cells with a wild-type β_2-microglobulin gene. Interestingly, the loss of MHC class I antigens via defective β_2-microglobulin expression can be induced by immunotherapy with IL-2, indicating that this mechanism is employed by tumor cells to escape from immune recognition when selective pressure is enhanced by immune modulation (63).

Recent studies have shown that a number of melanoma cell lines and several melanoma lesions can only be weakly stained by monoclonal antibodies to monomorphic determinants of MHC class I. Further characterization of one such cell line has shown that the level of MHC class I expression is enhanced by incubation with either interferon at 37°C or synthetic oligopeptides at 26°C. Pulse-chase experiments demonstrated that MHC class I molecules were not transported from the endoplasmatic reticulum to the cell surface in these cell lines (58). This suggested that peptides were not available for binding to nascent MHC molecules in the endoplasmatic reticulum. Further characterization of these cell lines revealed that they lack expression of the MHC-encoded proteasome or the transporter associated with antigen processing (64,65). However, Straten et al. have analyzed 38 melanoma cell lines for the expression of mRNA transcripts coding for such proteins, i.e., TAP 1/2 and LMP 2/7 (48). In this rather large number of cell lines, no loss of expression for any of these proteins could be detected.

Besides the loss or downregulation of all MHC class I antigens, there is also a selective downregulation of HLA-B antigens (66). Abrogation of HLA-B antigens is correlated with the overexpression of the c-myc oncogene (67). Furthermore, downregulation of HLA-B antigens was found on melanoma cells with low endogenous c-myc expression following transfection with the c-myc oncogene. Recent studies confirmed the regulatory role of the c-myc oncogene on MHC class I expression at the level of transcription. However, the main enhancer of the MHC class I genes (Enhancer A) is not involved in this process (67).

Analysis of expression of MHC class I allospecificities on melanoma is hampered by the availability of monoclonal antibodies to only a few allotypes. One of the allospecificities analyzed for altered expression is HLA-A2, which is particularly interesting since a number of oligopeptides derived from tumor antigens have been found to be presented by this MHC allotype. Selective loss of HLA-A2 antigens has been found in 25% of primary and 31% of metastatic melanoma lesions (66,68). The loss of class I allospecificities ranges from a full haplotype to an individual allele. It should be noted that both the down-regulation of only one class I locus, as well as the selective loss of class I allospecificities, did not significantly alter the staining patterns of antibodies directed against monomorphic determinants shared by HLA-A, -B, and -C antigens (58).

B. Modulation of T-Cell Responses

An individual T cell at any of the states of differentiation— i.e., naïve, primary effector, memory, or secondary effector—

can undergo one or more of a panel of responses when encountering an antigen via its TCR. Depending on the nature of the stimulus, cells can get fully activated, partially activated, or even anergized (15,16,69). These differential responses appear to reflect the particular signaling pathways which are triggered (28). Although such diverse reactions of T cells are necessary to avoid the development of autoimmune responses against normal tissues, they can be detrimental in the case of cancer. Indeed, T cells isolated from animals and patients with cancer may respond less well than those from healthy controls in vitro to immune stimuli, e.g., mitogens or recall antigens (70). Furthermore, patients with cancer often show poor delayed type hypersensitivity responses in vivo (71).

1. *Signal Transduction*

The molecular basis for this T-cell dysfunction in tumor bearing hosts is becoming better understood. There is increasing evidence that abnormalities in the signal transduction events of activated T cells are involved (72). These abnormalities include altered patterns of protein tyrosinase phosphorylation by PTKs, decreased protein levels of the PTK $p56^{lck}$ and $p59^{fyn}$, and of the CD3ζ chain, any of which could contribute to the development of the observed T-cell dysfunction (70,72–74). Furthermore, immunohistochemistry directly demonstrated the diminished ζ-chain expression in lymphocytes infiltrating into melanoma (A.C. Ochoa and T.L. Whiteside, presentations at the 2nd Tumor Immunology Forum: Mechanisms of Tumor Escape from Immune Recognition, Milan, April 1996). Even if normal protein concentrations of the CD3ζ chain and of the PTKs $p56^{lck}$ and $p59^{fyn}$ are present in such T cells, they still might display decreased protein tyrosine phosphorylation (75). A possible explanation for these observations might be the activation of $p50^{csk}$. Csk is a cytoplasmatic PTK with homology to Src-like kinases (32,76).

However, in contrast to Src-like kinases, p50[csk] lacks the amino-terminal myristylation signal or an inhibitory carboxy-terminal tyrosine phosphorylation site. Csk phosphorylates this negative regulatory carboxy-terminal tyrosine residue of PTKs of the src-family, e.g., p56[lck] and p59[fyn], with exquisite specificity. Preliminary results obtained in melanoma-bearing C57BL/6 mice suggest an increased p50[csk] protein concentration and activity in splenocytes and TIL as compared to normal controls (J.C. Becker and R.A. Reisfeld, unpublished results).

2. Transcriptional Regulation

The second possible molecular mechanisms for the observed T-cell dysfunction in tumor patients seems to be located directly on the level of gene transcription. Abnormalities in transcription factors of the NF-κB/Rel family have been described in T cells of tumor-bearing mice and TIL from renal-cell carcinomas and melanoma (77–79). We recently demonstrated that a CD4[+] T-cell clone that has been isolated from TIL and the autologous MHC class II[+] melanoma cell line interact with each other, which leads to an increase of $[Ca^{2+}]_i$ in the T-cell clone (79). However, this interaction failed to induce IL-2 production or proliferation of the T-cell clone, but rendered it unresponsive to subsequent stimulation. Transfection of the melanoma cells with an expression vector containing a CD80 cDNA altered the effect of this T-cell/melanoma interaction resulting in enhanced IL-2 transcription. Comparison of the amount of transcription factors binding to the IL-2 promoter—i.e., NF-AT1, Octamer, NFκB, AP-1, and CD28RC—during anergy induction or activation confirmed that induction members of the NFκB/Rel family are altered in anergic cells (80). Moreover, high amounts of a binding activity to the negative regulatory element A (NRE-A) of the IL-2 promoter were detected in nuclear extracts from human T cells shortly after induction of anergy. Rapid induction of this nuclear complex is blocked by cyclosporin A and is found to be independent of protein synthesis. Plasmid DNAs, containing either the human TPA responsive element (TRE) or both NRE-A and TRE, were used as template for in vitro transcription assays. Under these conditions, nuclear extracts obtained from both anergic and activated T-cell clones induced transcription of plasmids containing only TRE. However, when plasmids containing NRE-A and TRE were used, transcription was induced only by nuclear extracts from activated but not anergic T cells. These findings suggest the functional relevance of transcriptional repression of the IL-2 gene in anergic T cells.

C. Cytokines

Peptide-regulating factors, i.e. cytokines, are released spontaneously or upon stimulation by melanoma cells in culture (81–83). Among these cytokines are factors such as TGFβ1 and IL-10, which are basically acting as immune-regulatory molecules. One way melanoma cells are likely to modulate T-cell responses is by production of such cytokines.

TGFβ is a prototypical, multifunctional cytokine that was first isolated from platelets about ten years ago (84,85). In mammals, this cytokine has five isoforms whose biologic properties are nearly identical. TGFβ1 is synthesized as a 391-amino-acid precursor molecule and proteolytically cleaved to yield several peptide fragments and an 112-amino-acid subunit. It is secreted in an inactive form that requires activation before it can exert its biologic effects. Inactive TGFβ1 is stored at the cell surface and in the extracellular matrix and is converted to the active form at these sites (86). Overproduction of TGFβ has been found in a number of different neoplastic cells, including melanoma (85,87,88). One of the multiple advantages gained by tumor cells by an increased TGFβ1 synthesis is based on the ability of this cytokine to exert a local immunosuppressive effect, e.g., the inhibition of lymphocyte proliferation and cytotoxicity (89).

IL-10 was identified as another immune-suppressive cytokine possibly produced by melanoma cells (81,90). In vitro studies have demonstrated that IL-10 directly suppresses T cell proliferation by specific inhibition of IL-2 production and has potent inhibitory effects on allo-antigen induced proliferative and cytotoxic T-cell responses (91–93). Furthermore, IL-10 is able to suppress the innate immunity exerted by macrophages and NK cells. Overall, these biological activities of IL-10 indicate that it is a potent negative regulator of immunoproliferative and inflammatory responses.

The abnormal expression of growth factors has been correlated consistently with neoplastic transformation in human cells. In-situ studies demonstrate the production of negative regulatory cytokines in primary and metastatic melanoma (94). Moreover, significantly higher amounts of mRNA encoding for both TGFβ1 and IL-10 can be detected in tumor cells from progressing areas than are detected in those from regression zones of primary melanomas (C.T. Conrad and J.C. Becker, unpublished results). Tumor cell heterogeneity reflected in the production of these cytokine may contribute to a number of clinical features of melanoma, i.e., partial regression of the malignant tumor. Thus, while an efficient host immune response destroys susceptible tumor cell populations, tumor cells capable of inducing a local immune suppression proliferate in adjacent sites.

D. Intercellular Adhesion Molecule (ICAM-1)

Cell surface adhesion molecules are thought to play an important role in establishing the intercellular contacts that are essential for immunological reactions (95). One of these adhesion pathways in humans involves the β_2 leukocyte integrin LFA-1 (CD11a/CD18) and its ligand ICAM-1 (CD54). The ICAM-1 molecule has a M_r of 90,000 and is composed of five Ig-like extracellular domains, a hydrophobic transmembrane domain, and a short cytoplasmic domain. ICAM-1 is constitutively expressed or can be induced on a wide range of cells of hematopoietic and nonhematopoietic origin and tumor cells, including melanoma. ICAM-1 is induced or upregulated by proinflammatory cytokines such as IFNγ and TNF in vitro. In vivo it is not expressed in benign melanocytic nevi but occurs in proportion to local and systemic melanoma progression; thus it is regarded as a progression marker (5,96,97).

Cytolytic conjugates between CTLs and tumor cells are stabilized by LFA-1/ICAM-1 interactions (95). Lack of expression of ICAM-1 appears to permit circulating tumor cells to avoid establishing stable cytolytic conjugates and provides a means of evading T-cell-mediated killing. Paradoxically, as discussed above, progression toward metastasis in melanoma is accompanied by upregulated expression of ICAM-1 (5,96,97). However, the finding of soluble ICAM-1 in the sera of melanoma patients suggests that the release of this molecule by high-producing tumor cells may block its receptor (98,99). In this regard, it has been shown that soluble forms of cell surface macromolecules appear to compete with membrane-bound forms for binding to their ligands (100). Purified soluble ICAM-1 produced in CHO cells, as well as concentrated cell-free supernatants containing soluble ICAM-1 shed from a human melanoma cell line, inhibited T cell/melanoma conjugate formation and MHC-restricted cytotoxicity (101,102). Although the concentrations of soluble ICAM-1 detected in the serum of melanoma patients are not sufficient to block non-MHC-restricted cell–cell interactions, nothing is known about the concentrations of soluble ICAM-1 in the microenvironment of the tumor.

V. CONCLUSIONS

Human melanoma is an immunogenic tumor which is characterized by a number of defined tumor associated antigens and a specific T-cell mediated immune response. Nevertheless, there is only limited evidence for an effective anti-tumor immune response capable of eradicating established primary or secondary melanoma. This is due to the fact that melanoma cells have multiple avenues from host T-cell responses. Increasing the understanding of the cellular and molecular mechanisms of immune escape is likely to enable the development of more effective therapeutic strategies for melanoma patients.

ACKNOWLEDGMENT

This manuscript is dedicated in memoriam to our dear friend Stéphane Carrel.

REFERENCES

1. Becker JC, Schwinn A, Dummer R, Burg G, Bröcker EB. Lesion-specific activation of cloned tumor infiltrating lymphocytes by autologous tumor cells: induction of proliferation and cytokine production. J Invest Dermatol 1993; 101:15–21.
2. Boon T, Gajewski TF, Coulie PG. From defined human tumor antigens to effective immunization? Immunol Today 1995; 16:334–336.
3. Topalian S, Solomon D, Rosenberg SA. Tumor specific cytolysis by lymphocytes infiltrating human melanomas. J Immunol 142 (1989); 3714–3724.
4. Van den Eynde B, Hainaut P, Herin M, Knuth A, Lemoine C, Weynants P, van der Bruggen P, Fauchet R, Boon T. Presence on a human melanoma of multiple antigens recognized by autologous CTL. Int J Cancer 1989; 44:634–640.
5. Bröcker EB, Zwadlo G, Holzmann B, Macher E, Sorg C. Inflammatory cell infiltrates in human melanoma at different stages of tumor progression. Int J Cancer 1988; 41:562–567.
6. Tefany FJ, Barnetson,RS, Halliday GM, McCarthy SW, MacCarthy WH. Immunocytochemical analysis of the cellular in-

filtrate in primary regressing and non-regressing malignant melanoma. J Invest Dermatol 1991; 97:197–202.

7. Koh HK. Cutaneous Melanoma. N Eng J Med 1991; 171–182.

8. Kelly JW, Sagebiel RW, Blois MS. Regression in malignant melanoma. Cancer 1985; 56:2287–2291.

9. Ronan SG, Eng AM, Briele HA, Shioural NN, Gupta TKD. Thin malignant melanomas with regression and metastases. Arch Dermatol 1987; 123:1326–1330.

10. Carbone FR, Bevan MJ. Major histocompatibility complex control of T cell recognition, in W.E. Paul, ed. Fundamental Immunology. New York: Raven Press, 1989, 541–570.

11. Rammensee H-G, Rötzschke O, Falk K. MHC class I-restricted antigen processing. In: A. Sette, ed. Naturally processed peptides. Chemical Immunology Base: Karger, 1993, 113–133.

12. Goldberg AL, Rock KL. Proteolysis, proteasomes and antigen presentation. Nature 1992; 357:375–379.

13. Romagnoli P, Germain RN. Inhibition of invariant chain (Ii)-calnexin interaction results in enhanced degradation of Ii but does not prevent assembly of alpha Ii complexes. J Exp Med 1995; 182:2027–2036.

14. Urban RG, Chicz RM, Vignali DAA, Strominger JL. The dichotomy of peptide presentation by class I and class II MHC proteins. In: A. Sette, ed. Naturally processed peptides. Chemical Immunology. Basel: Karger, 1993, 197–234.

15. Allison JP. CD28-B7 interactions in T-cell activation. Curr Opin Immunol 1994; 6:414–419.

16. Sprent J. Professionals and amateurs. Curr Biol 1995; 5:1095–1097.

17. Kündig TM, Bachmann MF, DiPaolo C, Simrad JJL, Battegay M, Lother H, Gessner A, Kühlcke K, Ohashi PS, Henngartner H, Zinkernagel RM. Fibroblasts as efficient antigen-presenting cells in lymphoid organs. Science 1995; 268:1343–1347.

18. C.R. Mackay, T cell memory: the connection between function, phenotype, and migration pathways. Immunol Today 1991; 12:189–193.

19. Grant EP, Rock KL. MHC class I-restricted presentation of

exogenous antigen by thymic antigen presenting cells in vitro and in vivo. J Immunol 1992; 148:13–18.

20. Reis-e-Sousa C, Germain RN. Major histocompatibility complex class I presentation of peptides derived from soluble exogenous antigen by a subset of cells engaged in phagocytosis. J Exp Med 1995; 182:841–851.

21. Roche PA, Cresswell P. Invariant chain association with HLA-DR molecules inhibits immunogeneic peptide binding. Nature 1990; 345:615–618.

22. DeNagel DC, Pierce SK. A case for chaperones in antigen processing. Immunol Today 1992; 13:86–89.

23. Weissman AM. The T cell antigen receptor: a multisubunit signaling complex. In: Samelson, ed, *Lymphocyte activation*. Basel: Karger, 1993, 1–18.

24. Clothia C, Boswell DR, Lesk AM. The outline structure of the T-cell alpha beta receptor. EMBO J 1988; 7:3745–3755.

25. Davis MM, Bjorkman PJ. T-cell antigen receptor genes and T cell recognition. Nature 1988; 334:395–402.

26. Jorgensen JL, Esser U, Groth BF, Reay PA, Davis MM. Mapping T-cell receptor peptide contact by variant peptide immunization of single chain transgenics. Nature 1992; 355: 224–230.

27. Jin YL, Clayton LK, Howard FD, Koyasu S, Sieh M, Steinbrich R, Tarr GE, Reinherz EL. Molecular cloning of the CD3η subunit identifies a CD3 ζ-related product in thymus derived cells. Proc Natl Acad Sci USA 1990; 87: 3319–3323.

28. Weiss A, Littman DR. Signaltransduction by lymphocyte antigen receptors. Cell 1994; 6:263–274.

29. Iwashima M, Irving BA, van-Oers NS, Chan AC, Weiss A. Sequential interactions of TCR with two distinct cytoplasmatic tyrosine kinases. Science 1994; 263:1136–1139.

30. Chan AC, Iwashima M, Turck CW, Weiss A. ZAP-70: a 70 kD tyrosine kinase that associates with the TCR zeta chain. Cell 1992; 71:649–662.

31. Chu K, Littman DR. Requirement for kinase activity of CD4-associated p56lck in antibody-triggered T cell signal transduction. J Biol Chem 1994; 269:24095–24101.

32. Peri KG, Veillette A. Tyrosine protein kinases in T lympho-

cytes. In: L. E. Samelson, ed. Lymphocyte activation. Basel: Karger, 1993, 19–39.

33. Valitutti S, Muller S, Cella M, Paduvan E, Lanzavecchia, A. Serial triggerering of many T-cell receptors by a few peptide-MHC complexes. Nature 1995; 375:148–151.

34. Gulbins E, Schlottmann K, Brenner B, Lang F, Coggeshall K. Molecular analysis of ras activation by tyrosine phosphorylation Vav. Biochem Biophys Res Commun 1995; 217:876–885.

35. Fraser JD, Strauss D, Weiss A. Signal transduction events leading to T cell lymphokine gene expression. Immunol Today 1993; 14:357–61.

36. Fraser JD, Irving BA, Crabtree CR, Weiss A. Regulation of Interleukin-2 gene enhancer activity by the T cell accessory molecule CD28. Science 1991; 251:313–316.

37. Serfling E, Barthelmäs R, Pfeuffer I, Schenk B, Zarius S, Swoboda R, Mercurio F, Karin,M. Ubiquitous and lymphocyte-specific factors are involved in the induction of the mouse interleukin 2 gene in T lymphocytes. EMBO 1989; 8:465–73.

38. Seder RA, Germain RN, Linsley PS, Paul WE. CD28-mediated costimulation of interleukin 2 (IL-2) production plays a critical role in T cell priming for IL-4 and interferon gamma production. J Exp Med 1994; 179:299–304.

39. Ghosh P, Tan TH, Rice NR, Sica A, Young HA. The interleukin 2 CD28-responsive complex contains at least three members of the NF κB family: c-Rel, p50, and p65. Proc Nat Acad Science USA 1993; 90:1696–1700.

40. Darrow T, Slingluff C, Seigler H. The role of HLA class I antigens in recognition of melanoma cells by tumor-specific cytotoxic T lymphocytes: evidence for shared tumor antigens. J Immunol 1989; 142:3329–3335.

41. Sensi M, Parmiani G. Analysis of TCR usage in human tumors. Immunol Today 1995; 16:588–595.

42. Weidmann E, Elder EM, Trucco M, Lotze MT, Whiteside TL. Usage of T cell receptor V beta chain genes in fresh and cultured TIL from human melanoma. Int J Cancer 1993; 54:383–390.

43. thor-Straten P, Scholler J, Jensen KH, Zeuthen J. Preferential usage of T cell receptor alpha/beta variable regions

among tumor infiltrating lymphocytes in primary human malignant melanomas. Int. J. Cancer 1994; 56:78–86.

44. Sensi M, Salvi S, Castelli C, Maccalli C, Mazzocchi A, Mortarini R, Nicolini G, Herlyn M, Parmiani G, Anichini A. TCR structure of autologous melanoma-reactive CTL clones: TIL overexpress in vivo the TCR beta-chain sequence used by an HLA-A2-restricted and melanocyte-lineage-specific T cell clone. J Exp Med 1993; 178:1231–1246.

45. Salvi S, Segalla F, Rao S, Arienti F, Sartori M, Bratina G, Caronni E, Anichini A, Clemente C, Parmiani G. Overexpression of the T cell receptor beta-chain variable region TCRBV14 in HLA-A2-matched primary human melanomas. Cancer Res 1995; 55:3374–3379.

46. Coulie P, Brichard V, van-Pel A, Wölfel T, Schneider J, Traversari C, Mattei S, De-Plaen E, Lurquin C, Szikora JP, Renauld JC, Boon. A new genecoding for a differentiation antigen recognized by aurologous cytolytic T lymphoytes on HLA-A2 melanomas. J Exp Med 1994; 180:35–52.

47. Scholler J, thor-Straten P, Birck A, Siim E, Dahlstrom K, Zeuthen J. Analysis of T cell receptor alpha/beta variability in lymphocytes infiltrating melanoma primary tumors and metastatic lesions. Cancer Immunol Immunother 1994; 39:239–248.

48. thor-Straten P, Becker JC, Seremet T, Bröker EB, Zeuthen J. Clonal T cell responses in tumor infiltrating lymphocytes from both regressive and progressive regions of primary human malignant melanoma. J Clin Invest 1996 in press.

49. Boon T. Genetic analysis of tumor rejection antigens. Adv Cancer Res 1992; 58:177–210.

50. Chen YT, Stockert E, Tsang S, Coplan KA, Old LJ. Immunophenotyping of melanomas for tyrosinase: implications for vaccine development. Proc. Natl. Acad. Sci. USA 1995; 92:8125–8129.

51. Kawakami Y, Eliyahu S, Delgado CH, Robbins PF, Sakaguchi K, Appella E, Yannelli JR, Adema GJ, Miki T, Rosenberg, SA. Identification of a human melanoma antigen recognized by tumor-infiltrating lymphocytes associated with in vivo tumor rejection. Proc Natl Acad Sci USA 1994; 91:6458–6462.

52. Wang RF, Robbins PF, Kawakami Y, Kang XQ, Rosenberg, SA. Identification of a gene encoding a melanoma antigen recognized by HLA-A31-restricted tumor infiltrating lymphocytes. J Exp Med 1995; 181:799–804.

53. Traversari C, van der Bruggen P, Luescher IF, Lurquin C, Chomez P, Van PA, De PE, Amar CA, Boon T. A nonapeptide encoded by human gene MAGE-1 is recognized on HLA-A1 by cytolytic T lymphocytes directed against tumor antigen MZ2-E. J Exp Med 1992; 176:1453–1457.

54. Brasseur F, Marchand M, Vanwijck R, Herin M, Lethe B, Chomez P, and Boon T. Human gene MAGE-1, which codes for a tumor-rejection antigen, is expressed by some breast tumors [letter]. Int J Cancer 1992; 52:839–841.

55. Boel P, Wildmann C, Sensi ML, Brasseur R, Renauld JC, Coulie P, Boon T, van-der Bruggen P. BAGE: a new gene encoding an antigen recognized on human melanomas by cytolytic T lymphocytes. Immunity 1995; 2:167–175.

56. Wölfel T, Hauer M, Schneider, J, Serrano, M, Wölfel C, Klehmann-Hieb E, de-Plaen E, Hankeln T, Meyer-zum-Büschenfelde KH, Beach D. A p16INK4a-insensitive CDK4 mutant targeted by cytolytic T lymphocytes in a human melanoma. Science 1995; 269:1281–1284.

57. Carrido F, Cabrera T, Concha A, Glew S, Ruiz-Cabello F, Stern PL. Natural history of HLA expression during tumor development. Immunol Today 1993; 14:491–499.

58. Ferrone S, Marincola FM. Loss of HLA class I antigens by melanoma cells. Immunol Today 1995; 16:487–494.

59. Van-Duinen SG, Ruiter DJ, Broecker EB, Van-der-Velde EA, Sorg C, Welvaart K, Ferrone S. Level of HLA antigen in locoreginal metastases in clinical course of the disease in patients with melanoma. Cancer Res 1988; 48:1019–1025.

60. Carrel S, Dore JF, Ruiter DJ, Prade M, Lejeune FJ, Kleeberg UR, Rümke P, and Bröcker EB. The EORTC melanoma group exchange program: evaluation of a multicenter monoclonal antibody study. Int. J. Cancer 1991; 48:836–847.

61. D'Urso CM, Wang Z, Cao Y, Tatake R, Zeff RA, Ferrone S. Lack of HLA class I expression by cultured melanoma cells FO-1 due to a defect in beta2-microglobulin gene expression. J Invest Dermatol 1991; 87:284–292.

62. Wang Z, Cao Y, Albino AP, Zeff RA, Houghton A, Ferrone S. Lack of HLA class I antigen expression by melanoma cells SK-MEL-33 caused by a reading frameshift in beta2-microglobulin messenger RNA. J Clin Invest 1993; 91:684–692.
63. Restifo NP, Marincola FM, Kawakami Y, Taubenberger J, Yanenelli JR, Rosenberg, S.A. Loss of functional beta2-microglobulin in metastatic melanomas from five patients receiving immunotherapy. J Natl Cancer Inst 1996; 88:100–108.
64. Restifo NP, Esquivel F, Kawakami Y, Yewdell JW, Mule JJ, Rosenberg SA, Bennink JR. Identification of human cancers deficient in antigen processing. J Exp Med 1993; 177:265–272.
65. Cromme FV, Airey J, Haemels MT, Ploegh HL, Keating PJ, Stern PL, Meijer CJ, Walboomers JM. Loss of transporter protein, encoded by TAP-1 gene, is highly correlated with loss of HLA expression in cervical carcinomas. J Exp Med 1994; 179:335–340.
66. Marincola FM, Shamamian P, Alexander RB, Gnarra JR, Turetskaya RL, Nedospasov SA, Simonis TB, Taubenberger JK, Yannelli J, MA. Loss of HLA haplotype and B locus down regulation in melanoma cell lines. J Immunol 1994; 153:1225–1237.
67. Schrier PI, Peltenberg LTC. Relationship between myc oncogen activation and MHC class I expression. Adv Cancer Res 1993; 60:181–245.
68. Kageshita T, Wang Z, Calorini L, Yoshii A, Kimura T, Ono T, Gattoni-Celli S, Ferrone S. Selective loss of human leucocyte class I allospecificities and staining of melanoma cells by monoclonal antibodies recognizing monomorphic determinants of class I human leucocyte antigens. Cancer Res 1993; 53:3349–3354.
69. Swain SL. CD4 T cell development and cytokine polarzation: an overview. J Leukoc Biol 1995; 57:795–798.
70. Mizoguchi H, O'Shea JJ, Longo DL, Loeffler CM, McVicar DW, Ochoa AC. Alterations in signal transduction molecules in T lymphocytes from tumor bearing mice. Science 1992; 258:1795–1798.
71. Rünger TM, Klein CE, Becker JC, Bröcker, E-B-. The role of genetic instability, adhesion, cell motility, and immune es-

cape mechanisms in melanoma progression. Curr Opin Oncol 1994; 6:188–196.

72. Zier K, Gansbacher B, Salvadori S, preventing abnormalities in signal transduction of T cells in cancer: the promise of cytokine gene therapy. Immunol Today 1996; 17:39–45.

73. Nakagomi H, Petersson M, Magnusson I, Juhlin C, Matsuda M, Mellstedt H, Taupin JL, Vivier E, Anderson P, Kiessling R. Decreased expression of the signal-transducing zeta chains in tumor infiltrating T cells and NK cells of patients with colorectal carcinoma. Cancer Res 1993; 53: 5610–5612.

74. Finke JH, Zea AH, Stanley J, Longo DL, Mizoguchi H, Tubbs RR, Wiltout RH. Loss of T-cell receptor zeta chain and p56lck in T cells infiltrating human renal carcinoma. Cancer Res 1993; 53:5613–5616.

75. Wang Q, Stanley J, Kudoh S, Myles J, Kolenko V, Yi T, Tubbs R, Bukowski R, Finke J. T cells infiltrating non-Hodgkin's B cell lymphoma show altered tyrosine phosphorylation pattern even though T cell receptor/CD3-associated kinases are present. J Immunol 1995; 155:1382–1392.

76. Brauninger A, Karn T, Strebhardt K, Rubsamen-Waigmann H. Characterization of human CSK locus. Oncogene 1993; 8:1465–1469.

77. Ghosh P, Sica A, Young HA, Ye J, Franco JL, Wiltrout RH, Longo DL, Rice NR, Komschlies KL. Alterations in NF kappa B/rel family proteins in splenic T cells from tumor bearing mice and reversal following therapy. Cancer Res 1994; 54:2969–2972.

78. Li X, Liu J, Park JK, Hamilton TA, Rayman-P, Klein E, Edinger M, Tubbs R, Bukowski R, Finke J. T cells from renal cell carcinoma patients exhibit an abnormal pattern of kappa B-specific DNA binding activity. Cancer Res 1994; 54:5424–5429.

79. Becker JC, Brabletz T, Czerny C, Termeer C, Brocker EB. Tumor escape mechanisms from immunosurveillance: induction of unresponsiveness in a specific MHC-restricted CD4+ human T cell clone by the autologous MHC class II+ melanoma. Int Immunol 1993; 5:1501–1508.

80. Becker JC, Brabletz T, Kirchner T, Conrad CT, Bröcker EB,

Reisfeld RA. Negative transcriptional regulation in anergic T cells. Proc Natl Acad Sci USA 1995; 92:2375–2378.

81. Micksche M. Production of polypeptide regulatory factors by human melanoma cells. In vivo 1994; 8:859–865.

82. Mattei S, Colombo MP, Melani C, Silvani A, Parmiani G, Herlyn M. Expression of cytokine/growth factors and their receptors in human melanoma and melanocytes. Int J Cancer 1994; 56:853–857.

83. Dummer W, Becker JC, Schwaaf A, Leverkus M, Moll T, Bröcker EB. Elevated serum levels of interleukin 10 in patients with malignant melanoma. Mel Res 1995; 5:67–68.

84. Sporn MB, Roberts AB, Wakefield LM, Assoian RK. Transforming growth factor beta: biological function and chemical structure. Science 1986; 233:532–538.

85. Wahl S, M. Transforming growth factor beta: the good, the bad, and the ugly. J Exp Med 1994; 180:1587–1590.

86. Lyons RM, Gentry LE, Purchio AF, Moses HL. Mechanisms of activation of latent recombinant transforming growth factor beta1 by plasmin. J Cell Biol 1990; 110:1361–1367.

87. Reed JA, McNutt NS, Prieto VG, and Albino AP. Expression of transforming growth factor-beta2 in malignant melanoma correlates with the depth of tumor invasion. Am J Pathol 1994; 145:97–104.

88. Albino AP, Davis BM, and Nanus DM. Induction of growth factor RNA expression in human malignant melanoma: markers of transformation. Cancer Res 1991; 51:4815–4820.

89. Tada T, Ohzeki S, Utsumi K, Takiuchi H, Muramatsu M, Li XF, Shimizu J, Fujiwara H, Hamaoka T. Transforming growth factor beta-induced inhibition of T cell function: suceptibility difference in T cells of various phenotypes and functions and its relevance to immunosuppression in the tumor bearing state. J Immunol 1991; 146:1077–1082.

90. Chen P, Daniel V, Maher DW, Hersey P. Production of IL-10 by melanoma cells: examination of its role in immunosuppression mediated by melanoma. Int J Cancer 1994; 56:755–760.

91. Becker JC, Czerny C, Bröcker EB. Maintenance of clonal anergy by endogenously produced IL-10. Int Immunol 1994; 6:1605–1612.

92. deWaalMalefyt R, Yssel H, Roncarolo MG, Spits H, deVries JE. Interleukin-10. Curr Opin Immunol 1992; 4:314–321.
93. deWaalMalefyt R, Yssel H, deVries JE. Direct effects of IL-10 on subsets of human CD4+ T cell clones and resting T cells: specific inhibition of IL-2 production and proliferation. J Immunol 1993; 150:4754–4762.
94. Dummer W, Bastian B, Ernst N, Schänzle C, Schwaaf A, Bröcker EB, IL10 production in malignant melanoma: preferential detection of IL-10-secreting melanoma cells in metastatic lesions. Int J Cancer 1996; in press.
95. Springer TA. Adhesion receptors of the immune system. Nature 1990; 346:425–434.
96. Si Z, Hersey P. Immunohistological examination of the relationship between metastatic potential and expression of adhesion molecules and selectins on melanoma cells. Pathology 1994; 26:6–15.
97. Natali P, Nicotra MR, Cavaliere R, Bigotti A, Romano G, Temponi M, Ferrone S. Differential expression of ICAM-1 in primary and metastatic lesions. Cancer Res 1990; 50:1271–1278.
98. Kageshita T, Yoshii A, Kimura T, Kuriya N, Ono T, Tsujisaki M, Imai K, Ferrone S. Clinical relevance of ICAM-1 expression in primary lesions and serum of patients with malignant melanoma. Cancer Res 1993; 53:4927–4932.
99. Altomonte M, Colizzi F, Esposito G, Maio M. Circulating ICAM-1 as a marker of disease progression in cutaneous melanoma. N Eng J Med 1992; 327:959.
100. Gearing AJH, Newman W. Circulating adhesion molecules in disease. Immunol Today 1993; 14:506–512.
101. Becker JC, Dummer R, Hartmann AA, Burg G, Schmidt RE. Shedding of ICAM-1 from human melanoma cell lines induced by IFN-gamma and tumor necrosis factor-alpha. Functional consequences on cell-mediated cytotoxicity. J Immunol 1991; 147:4398–401.
102. Becker JC, Termeer C, Schmidt RE, Bröcker EB. Soluble intercellular adhesion molecule-1 inhibits MHC-restricted specific T cell/tumor interaction. J Immunol 1993; 151:7224–7232.

Part II
The Precursor Lesion in Melanoma
PROSPECTS FOR PREVENTION

3

COMMON ACQUIRED NEVI AND DYSPLASTIC NEVI AS PRECURSOR LESIONS AND RISK MARKERS OF MELANOMA

John T. Seykora and David E. Elder

University of Pennsylvania Medical Center
Philadelphia, Pennsylvania

I. INTRODUCTION

Melanocytic nevi and especially dysplastic nevi are potential simulants and risk markers of melanoma, and their role as harbingers of malignant disease warrants their recognition and appropriate management. Given that tumor progression is a variable temporal evolution of events along molecular, histologic, or clinical lines, the categorization of individual lesions may sometimes be difficult. Nevertheless, the concepts of dysplasia and of in situ as well as microinvasive malignancy are important steps in the classification of intermediate lesions of tumor progression. Conceptually, these lesions are clearly separable from early and late lesions and from one another, and there is evidence that criteria distinguishing them can be reproducibly applied. Analysis of these "intermediate lesions" suggests that they represent responses to events (probably mutational) that are either inherited or induced by ultraviolet light in constitutionally hypersensitive individuals, supporting epidemiological data that implicate genetics and sunlight as etiologic agents for some melanomas. The continuing rigorous application of the methodologies of epidemiology and basic science to the study of these lesional steps will lead to the recognition of biologic markers that distinguish benignancy from malignancy better than the presently available, solely morphologic criteria.

II. TUMOR PROGRESSION

Tumor progression, the "process whereby tumors go from bad to worse," was described by Foulds in terms of several principles: progression does not always reach the endpoint of metastasis within the lifetime of the host; the statistical chance of neoplastic development is greater in "precursor" lesions than in normal tissue (1,2). Foulds experienced great difficulty in naming these problematical precursor lesions. In his treatise

"Neoplastic Development," Foulds provisionally termed these lesions "Group B," intermediate between benign "Group A" and malignant "Group C" lesions. Likewise, Clark classified the steps of primary neoplasia as Classes I through III (3). Class I or "precursor" lesions, such as melanocytic nevi are characterized by stability, indolence, or regression, except for those rare lesions that progress to the next step. Within Clark's schema, melanocytic nevi with an abnormal pattern of intraepidermal melanocytic growth are classified as Class IB, and melanocytic nevi with dysplasia are categorized as Class IC (B1 lesions of Foulds). The Class II lesions termed "intermediate" in the Clark model are melanoma in situ and radial growth phase melanoma (nontumorigenic or microinvasive melanoma (4); these correspond to the B2 lesions of Foulds. These lesions are confined to the tissue compartment of origin, but their growth is not temporally restricted. Class III lesions, the C lesions of Foulds, are temporally unrestricted in growth, grow in two or more tissue compartments, and may have competence for metastasis, such as melanomas with a vertical growth phase (invasive and tumorigenic melanoma [4]).

The graph in Fig. 1 is adapted from the model of stepwise tumor progression. The slope of the lesion line in relationship to the time axis (*x*-axis) indicates Foulds's interest in the time dependency of increasing neoplastic capacity in any given system.

If one were to draw the vertical lines of Figure 1 with arrow lengths proportional to the number of lesions, the numbers of "A" lesions (nevi) might exdeed C2 (melanoma) by a factor of as much as 500,000, exemplifying the clinical observation that the vast majority of nevi (including dysplastic nevi) are stable lesions that do not progress to melanoma.

Molecular and Mathematical Models of Tumor Progression

Mathematical models for tumor development lead to a rational approach to quantitative cancer risk assessment and

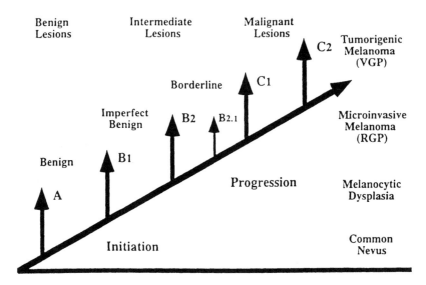

FIGURE 1 Stepwise tumor progression based on a model of Foulds. (Ref. 2.)

raise fundamental questions about the events leading to malignancy (5). Several studies have concluded that most cancers arise after four to seven steps (6–8). This is similar to the number of steps suggested by traditional morphology, reviewed above. A two-mutation model of carcinogenesis proposed by Moolgavkar and Knudsen, in which "intermediate cells" arising from "stem cells" eventually progress to "malignant cells," supports the idea of recessive oncogenesis (9). After malignant transformation, additional genetic or epigenetic events may contribute to the rate and extent of continuing tumor progression. If these concepts are valid, promoting agents—such as estrogens in breast cancer, cigarette smoke in lung cancer, or ultraviolet light in melanoma—may play an important role in human carcinogenesis by influencing the kinetics of intermediate lesions.

Molecular genetic analysis of human and animal neoplasms also provides compelling evidence for stepwise lesional tumor progression driven by a series of mutational events. The best-studied model is that of colorectal carcinogenesis. Vogelstein et. al. have demonstrated that colorectal cancers arise as a result of mutational changes that activate oncogenes and cause the functional loss of tumor-suppressor genes (10). These studies have established that mutations of at least four to five genes are necessary to generate a malignant tumor (carcinoma), while fewer changes are required to form a benign tumor (adenoma). Here the best, characterized oncogene mutation involves the ras oncogene and appears to occur in a single cell of a pre-existing small adenoma, acting to produce a larger and more dysplastic tumor through clonal expansion.

III. MELANOCYTIC NEVI IN TUMOR PROGRESSION

Except for cosmetic significance, melanocytic nevi are important only for their relation to melanoma. We shall review evidence that nevi and especially dysplastic nevi are important simulants of melanoma, potential precursors of melanoma, and markers of increased risk for melanoma.

A useful definition of a melanocytic nevus is "a localized area of skin in which the pigment cells show persistent abnormalities of behavior affecting their growth, their population density, their morphology, and their melanogenesis" (11). This definition distinguishes nevus cells from melanocytes, which are normally solitary dendritic cells whose bodies are separated by those of intervening keratinocytes (12). Clinically, nevi are focal areas of hyperpigmentation, and, histologically, they present as a focal area of increased melanocytic cellularity.

A. Common Acquired Nevi

Melanocytic nevi may be regarded as benign neoplasms of melanocytes, though studies of clonality to satisfy the neoplastic hypothesis have not yet been done. Nevi are almost ubiquitous in humans, first appearing in early childhood and reaching a maximum in young adults (13). Thereafter, the number of nevi declines in older age groups (14). Three processes might account for this phenomenon. There is evidence from serial studies that some nevi disappear, either by a process of maturation and/or senescence/atrophy (15,16) or by a process akin to immunologic regression (17). The regression of common acquired nevi by a process of differentiation may be a part of neoplastic biology, as it is present in most, if not all neoplastic systems (3,18–20).

There is evidence that sunlight is a major etiologic factor for nevi. From studies of migrant laborers, it appears that sun exposure in the first 10 years of life is especially important (21). In a major case-control study of schoolchildren in Vancouver, risk factors for nevi were similar to those for melanoma, including sun exposure and sun susceptibility factors (13). Studies of nevi in twins indicate that there may be a strong inherited basis for total nevus count and hence melanoma risk, perhaps involving a number of interacting genes (22).

Abundant clinical and anecdotal evidence [reviewed in part below and previously (23)] indicates that nevi may be potential precursors of melanoma, though the frequency of such progression is very low. The total number of nevi is also one of the strongest risk factors for malignant melanoma (24), and nevi are also major potential simulants of melanoma. Most common nevi pose few if any difficulties of interpretation, but as nevi acquire atypical features, accurate diagnosis becomes more difficult, and the reproducibility of diagnosis falls.

B. Dysplastic Nevi

In 1978, Clark et al. published an account of two familial melanoma kindreds, describing special melanocytic nevi that were common among family members (25,26); these lesions were initially named "BK moles." Referring to Clark's work, Lynch et al. published a similar kindred in 1978, introducing the term "familial atypical multiple mole melanoma syndrome (FAMMM)" (27). In 1980, the term "dysplastic nevi" was applied because the lesions were clinically atypical and characterized by histologically immature and cytologically atypical patterns of nevus cells (28).

The earliest studies of dysplastic nevi were in hereditary melanoma kindreds. In 1980, Elder et al. reported similar lesions in nonfamilial ("sporadic" or "random") melanoma patients (29). Subsequently, case-control studies demonstrated that similar lesions occurred in individuals who neither had melanoma nor were members of hereditary melanoma kindreds (14,24,30–34). In 1983, dysplastic nevi were classified based on family history of melanoma and dysplastic nevi (35); the relative risk for melanoma ranged from a low risk in patients with dysplastic nevi without a family or personal history of melanoma (type A), to highest risk in patients with dysplastic nevi and a history of melanoma in two family members (type D-2). In the same year, an NIH consensus conference discussed precursor lesions of melanoma, and a consensus definition of "dysplastic nevus" was proposed (36). However, the term FAMMM continued to be used by several groups (37,38). Other groups introduced the term "clinically atypical nevus," arguing that "dysplasia" implied a histologic correlation which was neither always available nor necessary (32,39,40). In this review, we shall use the term "dysplastic nevi."

1. Clinical Features of Dysplastic Nevi

Clinical features of atypical (dysplastic) nevi discussed in early reports include considerations of size, profile, border, and color variegation (25,29,41). The morphology has been well illustrated (42–44). Dysplastic nevi were defined as lesions greater than 5 mm in diameter with a macular component by definition; a papule, if present, is usually located in the center of an ovoid macule, and the lesions are generally symmetrical. Border characteristics are very important, and while the border is usually fairly regular, it is characteristically ill-defined about all or a part of its circumference. The lesions are usually brown or tan, with some variegation of hue and depth, but without black in most cases. Pink colors are often present, which may be related to dermal inflammation but perhaps also to excess red pheomelanin relative to brown eumelanin pigment (45). Substantial asymmetry, excessive pigmentary variegation, and focal black areas or gray areas suggestive of partial regression should prompt a biopsy to rule out melanoma (42–44).

2. Histological Features of Dysplastic Nevi

The histological features of dysplastic nevi (clinically atypical nevi) in hereditary melanoma kindreds were described early by Clark et al. and subsequently have been reviewed (44). In summary, the three salient histologic features of dysplastic nevi are the presence of an immature or disordered pattern of growth, of focal ("random") cytologic atypia in melanocytes, and of a lymphocytic host response. High-grade or uniform cytologic atypia, pagetoid proliferation of atypical cells in the epidermis, and lesional cell mitoses are generally not observed; their presence should suggest consideration of the possibility of melanoma.

C. Nevi and Dysplastic Nevi as Potential Precursors of Melanoma

As discussed earlier, the significance of intermediate lesions as simulants and risk markers for cancer is related to their role as potential precursor lesions for cancer. Potential precursors are lesions within which the rate of cancer development is greater than that of normal tissue. Progression is not obligate and most potential precursors are stable within the lifetime of the host. Kraemer et al, have estimated that, even in the highest-risk patient populations, the lifetime risk of progression is of the order of one melanoma occurring in several hundred nevi (46). Individuals and populations with potential precursor lesions have an increased risk of cancer because cancers develop within some of the precursors and also because of shared risk factors (13).

The evidence that nevi and dysplastic nevi are potential precursors of melanoma is primarily histologic and usually inferential, because the rarity of progression in nevi has generally precluded direct observation. However, with the registration of patients for follow-up after initial photographic documentation of nevi, instances of evolution of melanomas from precursor nevi have been documented. In our experience, the evolution of melanoma within a precursor nevus generally presents as a small focus of darker pigment that expands within the precursor lesion, often completely replacing it. In contrast, melanomas without a precursor lesion typically demonstrate uniform changes of color, topography, and border that are global throughout the lesions as they grow from smaller to larger macules, patches, or nodules. While photographic and histologic evidence demonstrates melanoma arising in contiguity with nevi, an alternative explanation is that the association occurs by chance, or that some lesions interpreted as nevic precursors are actually nevocytically differentiated melanoma cells.

Large studies of the relationship between nevi and melanomas have been published (see Table 1). Between 5 and 39% (median 22%) of melanomas exhibit a contiguous dysplastic nevus, and banal (dermal) nevic cells are present in an additional 10–21% (median 15%) of cases. The incidence of a putative precursor nevus appears to be higher in relation to melanomas in high-risk populations and to melanomas that are diagnosed in surveillance programs (47,48).

TABLE 1

Incidence of Nevi in Contiguity with Melanomas

Study	Number of melanomas	Banal nevus	Histologic dysplasia	Any nevus
Rhodes et al. (49)[a]	225	—	22%	40%
Clark et al. (18)[a]	150	21%	39%	60%
McGovern et al. (50)	723	—	39%	—
Cook and Robertson (50)[b]	226	—	27%	—
Maize and Ackerman (51)	n.s.[c]	—	5%	—
English et al. (52)	117	—	22%	—
Black (53)	500	10%	32%	—
Hastrup et al. (54)	512	—	7%	—
Gruber et al. (55)	248	15%	17%	32%

[a]Superficial spreading melanomas only.
[b]Includes in situ cases.
[c]Not stated.

D.   Nevi and Dysplastic Nevi as Simulants of Melanoma

As some nevus cells progress along the steps of tumor progression, it is expected that they will acquire the molecular and morphologic attributes intermediate between common nevi and early melanomas and therefore become high-grade simulants of melanoma. The difficult distinctions among benign nevi, intermediate lesions, and other melanoma simulants such as spindle and epithelioid cell nevi, and melanomas have been well documented (56,57). The gold standard for ruling out melanoma in a clinically atypical lesion is excisional biopsy and histological examination.

Clinically dysplastic nevi and invasive melanomas are markers of risk for subsequent melanomas (58); as well, histologic dysplasia is associated with increased risk of melanoma in clinically selected lesions (59,60). It should be recognized that neither histologic severe dysplasia nor histologic melanoma in situ has been formally correlated with melanoma

risk in cohort or case-control studies. Thus, although a histologic diagnosis of dysplastic nevus should prompt a review of
other nevi and a detailed family history, the gold standard for
assessment of melanoma risk factors is the clinical evaluation
of nevi and other risk factors within the context of a family history, coupled with a consideration of behavioral attributes,
knowledge of skin cancer, and an environmental history.

E. Nevi and Dysplastic Nevi as Epidemiological Risk Factors for Melanoma

The significance of nevi as markers of individuals at increased risk for melanoma has been evaluated by two epidemiological methods: cohort and case-control studies. The
various studies have considered unselected nevi, typical nevi,
and/or dysplastic nevi. A few studies also have considered
histologic dysplasia, and some studies have incorporated a
requirement for histologic confirmation of a diagnosis of clinically dysplastic nevus. The cases usually have been drawn
from specialty clinics but occasionally from population-based
registries, as have the control groups.

1. Case-Control Studies in "Random" Melanoma

Case-control studies, by comparing prevalences in patients
with melanoma (cases) with those in controls, have established
that nevi and clinically dysplastic nevi are associated with increased risk for melanoma in people who are not members of
hereditary melanoma kindreds (see Table 2). These studies
have shown that dysplastic nevi are relatively common in the
community, their incidence ranging from 5 to 20% (median
13%). Other risk markers identified in case-control studies
have included total number of nevi (14,24,61), the presence and
number of freckles (32), the number of large nevi, a derivative
of nevus number and size called total nevus density (62,63),
quantitative history of sunburn (64), and sometimes other
markers of sun exposure or susceptibility. In every case-control

TABLE 2

Relative Risk Estimates for Common and Dysplastic Nevi

Study	Adjusted Relative Risks	
	Common nevi	Dysplastic nevi
Nordlund et al. (31); Australia	—	7.7 (any dysplastic nevi)
Holly et al. (24); San Francisco	4.4 (26–50 nevi) 6.2 (51–100 nevi)	3.8 (1–5 dysplastic nevi) 6.3 (6+ dysplastic nevi)
Garbe et al. (34); Germany	7.3 (41–60 nevi) 14.7 (>60 nevi)	11.4 (1–2 atypical nevi) 6.0 (>2 atypical nevi)
MacKie et al. (65); Glasgow	6.7 (>20 nevi)	2.1 (1–2 atypical nevi) 4.4 (3+ atypical nevi)
Halpern et al. (14); Pennsylvania	6.5 (>25 nevi)	6.8 (any dysplastic nevi)
Augustsson et al. (60); Stockholm	1.4 (75–149 nevi) 3.9 (>149 nevi)	2.5 (1–2 dysplastic nevi) 15.6 (>2 dysplastic nevi) 4.6 (histologic dysplasia)

study reported, the relative risk for melanoma is increased in patients who have clinically dysplastic nevi, and this risk persists after adjustment for the total number of nevi and other risk factors. The relative risk estimates for common nevi and dysplastic nevi are presented in Table 2. These estimates, from different continents and time periods, are remarkably consistent for both common nevi and dysplastic nevi as independent traits. Most studies have demonstrated a dose-response relationship for dysplastic and common nevi with risk for melanoma, and some studies have demonstrated a similar trend for increasing numbers of dysplastic nevi.

Most of the case-control studies presented in Table 2 have been based on analysis of the clinical phenotype (clinically atypical or dysplastic nevi). Some have also incorporated a biopsy component for some patients and/or controls. In Augustsson's study (60), a relative risk of 4.6 was determined for histologic dysplasia based on pattern criteria in which cytologic atypia of significant degree was "usually not seen." Thus, none of these case-control studies was designed to assess the particular contribution of cytologic atypia to melanoma risk assessment. Further, these studies have in some cases established a relation between risk and the number of dysplastic nevi, but the degree of clinical atypia has not been correlated with risk or with the degree of histological atypia. All of the studies have adjusted for total number of nevi in assessing the risk for dysplastic nevi and have therefore concluded that the two traits are independent risk markers (66).

The consistency of the risk estimates for dysplastic nevi in Table 2 is remarkable because diagnostic criteria were not uniform among the studies. Variation in the prevalence of nevi in the case and control populations among the studies may be related in large measure to this diagnostic heterogeneity. Studies using less specific and thus more sensitive criteria appear to have determined higher prevalence estimates for dysplastic nevi in their respective communities (see Table 3). Note that in the last three studies listed, with an average population prevalence more than twice that of the first three studies, papular compound nevi could have qualified as "dysplastic" if they were 5 mm in diameter and had pigmentary variegation including pink hues. In our view, the presence of a macular component is an essential element of the criteria for "clinically atypical (dysplastic) nevus."

2.   Cohort Studies in "Random" and Hereditary Melanoma

After the recognition of dysplastic nevi, an eight-year cohort study of familial melanoma, kindreds with two or more melanomas, was conducted by Greene and colleagues (47). Melanoma risk was transmitted as an autosomal dominant hereditary trait (67), closely related to cutaneous dysplastic nevi (47). In this prospective cohort study, 401 members of 14

TABLE 3

Criteria and Prevalence Estimates of Dysplastic Nevi

Study	Criteria	Prevalence
Nordlund et al. (31,66)	Size >5 mm, with an irregular border and haphazard color	5%
Garbe et al. (34)	Three of: size >5 mm, undefined border, irregular margin, color variegation, papular and macular components	5%
Halpern et al. (14)	All of: size >4 mm, macular component, color variegation, ill-defined and/or irregular margin	9%
Holly et al. (24)	Three of: size >5 mm, ill-defined border, irregular pigment, erythema, irregular border, accentuated skin markings	17%
Augustsson et al. (60)	>5 mm and two of: ill-defined border, speckled pigment, erythema, pebbled surface	18%
MacKie et al. (65)	>5 mm and one of: irregular edge, areas of inflammation, irregular pigmentation	20%

hereditary melanoma kindreds were followed for eight years, during which time 39 newly diagnosed melanomas occurred in 22 family members at first examination or in follow-up. The new melanomas occurred only in family members with dysplastic (clinically atypical) nevi. The actuarial probability of the development of melanoma in family members with dysplastic nevi was 56.0% from age 20 to age 59, while the prospective risk for members without dysplastic nevi was normal. This study has been recently updated and now comprises 23 kindreds. Forty-seven melanomas have occurred prospectively, all in family members with dysplastic nevi.

The cumulative risk by age 50 among family members with dysplastic nevi was 48.9%, and the risk of developing melanoma was increased 85-fold in family members with dysplastic nevi (68). These findings were confirmed in a data set of 311 families by Carey et al. who found dysplastic nevi and a prior history of melanoma to be strong risk factors for (additional) melanomas in these kindreds (69).

These findings have been confirmed by cohort studies that have included patients from hereditary and random kindreds. Rigel et al. followed 452 patients with dysplastic nevi classified into risk groups according to history of melanoma (70). They detected 18 newly diagnosed melanomas during an average follow-up period of 27 months. Risk was increased in all groups but was greater in patients with prior personal or family histories of melanoma. Halpern et al. reported on the follow-up of 153 patients over an average of 94 months (58). Eleven new melanomas had developed in eleven individuals for an age-adjusted incidence of 692 per 100,000 person-years, approximately 70 times the expected rate for an unselected population. The development of melanoma was strongly correlated with a prior personal and family history of melanoma (see Table 4). The incidence of melanoma in patients with dysplastic nevi but no history of melanoma was also increased, about 15 times more than population rates. Several studies have thus demonstrated that dysplastic nevi are a major independent risk factor for subsequent primary melanoma in individuals who have had prior melanoma, suggesting the need for lifelong cutaneous surveillance (69,71–75).

The cohort studies, as well as other studies of familial melanoma kindreds (48), have demonstrated that most melanomas detected in surveillance studies are early lesions, for which cure can confidently be expected by simple therapy. Thus, the recognition of clinically dysplastic nevi permits focused efforts in patient education and surveillance of high-risk groups.

TABLE 4
Incidence Rates of Melanoma in Follow-up
of Dysplastic Nevus Cases

Personal history of melanoma	Total melanomas in family	Crude incidence rate	Age-adjusted incidence rate[a]
Unselected Pennsylvania residents		9.7	9.7
Negative	0 or 1	295	154
Positive	1	1,479	968
Negative	≥2	2,838	1,955
Positive	≥2	2,966	12,313

[a]Rates were standardized to the 1985 Pennsylvania population using the direct method. 1985 Pennsylvania (white) overall melanoma incidence = 9.7/100,000.
Source: Ref. 58.

IV. NEVI AND DYSPLASTIC NEVI IN A MODEL OF TUMOR PROGRESSION

Clinical and laboratory studies of nevi have contributed much new information about the developmental biology of cancer. Studies of potential precursor lesions promise to elucidate the biological mechanisms of steps of tumor progression from a precursor nevus to melanoma. Studies of host biology address factors that contribute to the significance of intermediate lesions as markers of melanoma risk. These studies include investigations of host cellular factors, such as pigmentation or DNA repair mechanisms that may influence the susceptibility of lesional as well as nonlesional tissue to etiologic agents, and the genetic analysis of pedigrees at high risk for melanoma.

A. Cell Biology of Nevi and Dysplastic Nevi

If potential precursor lesional cells undergo progression, they acquire biological properties of cancer in a stepwise fashion.

These changes presumably result from mutations of various genes as well as epigenetic processes such as DNA methylation changes (76). The high-grade simulants (dysplasias) and early lesions of cancer are important for evaluating changes in genes and gene products that result in malignant behavior. Numerous studies of the biology of atypical and dysplastic nevi have now been published. In sum, these studies demonstrated biological properties intermediate between those of banal nevi and melanomas.

Several studies have explored the immunohistological profile of histologically dysplastic nevi. In a study of 14 potential tumor progression antigens, Elder et al. found that the reactivity of dysplastic nevus cells and cells of radial growth phase melanomas was intermediate between mature dermal nevus cells and cells of tumorigenic vertical growth-phase melanomas for several antigens, including gangliosides GD2 and GD3, and the epidermal growth factor receptor (77). Similarly, Ruiter et al. described an antibody to the transferrin receptor, PAL-M1, which reacted with 2/26 common nevi, 9/35 dysplastic nevi, and 14/19 primary melanomas, placing dysplastic nevi in an intermediate position (78,79). Taken together, these data are consistent with the hypothesis that histologically dysplastic nevi are intermediate lesions of tumor progression between banal lesions and melanomas. The progression antigens mentioned above may have significance in the development of the neoplastic phenotype of the intermediate lesions.

Jimbow et al. have described a series of human melanosome-associated (HMSA) antibodies associated with tumor progression in histologically dysplastic nevi. Melanosomes in these lesions exhibit alterations in the fine structure of the melanosomal matrix and in the pattern of melanization. The monoclonal antibodies HMSA-1 and HMSA-2 identify a structural matrix protein unique to melanosomes of neoplastic melanocytes that is present in epidermal dysplastic melanocytes and melanoma cells but not in epidermal melanocytes of most common nevi (80,81). Jimbow's group also demonstrated an increasing content of the red pheomelanin pigment at the expense of brown eumelanin, from normal skin to common nevi, then to dysplastic nevi, and finally to melanoma. There was "a much higher content of pheomelanin in dysplastic nevi compared to common nevi" (82). Pheomelanin has been shown to generate toxic superoxide radicals after UV exposure (83), and UV-irradiated pheomelanin can induce mutagenesis (84).

These observations suggest a mechanism of phototoxic insult resulting in DNA damage that could constitute a basis for the postulated precursor role of dysplastic nevi. Direct evidence for damage to the DNA in dysplastic nevi has been provided by Parmiter et al., who observed chromosomal translocations in 0/24 common nevi but 2/10 dysplastic nevi (85). In the morphometric studies of Schmiegelow et al., dysplastic nevus cells differed from those of common nevi in nuclear area, coefficient of variability (anisokaryosis), and DNA content (86). Similarly, Santucci et al. found by morphometry of nuclear area, perimeter, and form factor that "median values turned out to be intermediate between those of common acquired nevi and those of melanomas" (87). These authors emphasized the importance of atypical melanocytes in the diagnosis of melanocytic dysplasia. These findings are consistent with the hypothesis that tumor progression in nevi results in the accumulation of DNA damage and in the progressive appearance of cytologic atypia.

B. Host Cellular and Molecular Biology

Patients with atypical or dysplastic nevi exhibit biological markers in somatic and/or lesional cells, including abnormalities of DNA repair and evidence of hypermutability. These abnormalities provide a biologic basis for the increased melanoma risk in these patients.

1. Hypersensitivity to Ultraviolet Light

Studies have demonstrated abnormal responses of somatic cells to UV light in patients with dysplastic nevi. Early studies demonstrated an increased sensitivity of fibroblasts to UV killing (88). Two subsequent studies demonstrated increased sister chromatid exchanges after UV exposure in lymphoblastoid cells (89,90). Kraemer's laboratory demonstrated increased mutations induced by UV light in the cells of patients with dysplastic nevi (91). Roth et al. demonstrated an abnormal rate of repair in the first 60 minutes after UV-induced DNA damage to fibroblasts in seven out of eight patients with dysplastic nevi (92). Repair rates after 60 minutes were normal, suggesting an abnormality of the early phase of repair of UV-damaged DNA. This is consistent with Sanford et al.'s observation of increased chromatid damage in cells from patients with dysplastic nevi after exposure of cultures synchronized in the premitotic G2 phase of the cell cycle to UV light (93). In an important recent study, Hürlimann et al. were able to identify family members affected by dysplastic nevi by measuring the UVB- and UVC-driven increase in sister chromatid exchange (SCE), a measure related to hypermutability. A patient with melanoma and his son and nephew with dysplastic nevi all showed a distinctive elevation of UV-induced SCE, while four unaffected members of the family showed normal values (94). These authors conclude that, in a family with dysplastic nevi, the syndrome carrier can be well identified not only at the clinicopathologic level but also at the cytogenetic level by the elevation of SCE per millijoule of UV.

In an Australian study, analyses of familial and sporadic melanoma cell lines for p16 mutations, a tumor-suppressor gene to be discussed in more detail below, demonstrated a high frequency of C:G to T:A transitions often occurring at dipyrimidine sites. These lesions are characteristic of UV-induced mutations. Thus, this study links UV-induced mutagenesis and DNA hypermutability with melanoma-genesis (95).

Given the DNA fragility and hypermutability reviewed above, it is not surprising that cells from patients with dysplastic nevi show an increased incidence of chromosomal abnormalities compared to those of controls (85,90,96,97), suggesting that these patients may have a form of chromosomal instability (85). These data are consistent with the hypothesis that changes in cellular DNA induced by ultraviolet light are important in melanoma development, and that some of these changes may occur in nevi, especially atypical or dysplastic nevi. The findings are also consistent with the nuclear abnormalities and disordered patterns of growth in dysplastic nevi, and with the epidemiologic evidence implicating these lesions as risk markers, potential precursors, and morphologically intermediate lesions of tumor progression.

2. Molecular and Cell Biology of Intermediate Lesions in a Tumor Progression Model

Molecular genetic analysis of human and animal neoplasms also provides compelling evidence for stepwise lesional tumor progression driven by a series of mutational events. The best studied model is that of colorectal carcinogenesis. Fearon and Vogelstein have demonstrated that colorectal cancers arise as a result of mutational changes that activate oncogenes and/or cause the functional loss of tumor-suppressor genes (10). These studies have established that mutations of at least four to five genes are necessary to generate a malignant tumor (carcinoma), while fewer changes are required to form a benign tumor (adenoma). Considering five major genetic alterations of oncogenes and suppressor genes, Fearon and Vogelstein proposed a five-step model of progression from normal epithelium through hyperproliferative epithelium, to early, intermediate, and late adenomas, to carcinoma. In this model, the lesions termed early, intermediate, and late adenomas represent tumors of "increasing size, dysplasia and villous content." Here, the best characterized oncogene mutation involves the ras oncogene and appears to occur in a single cell of a pre-existing small adenoma, acting to produce a larger and more dysplastic tumor through clonal expansion. Such multistep mutational models of tumorigenesis probably exist in most, if not all, organ systems, and they probably account for many of the lesions that are clinically evaluated.

Recent studies have indicated that p16 (INK4a), a cyclin-dependent kinase inhibitor, is mutated in melanoma cell lines and familial melanoma. A study by Fountain et al. reported loss of heterozygosity at 9p21 in multiple melanoma tumors and cell lines; this study provided evidence that a tumor-suppresser gene associated with melanoma is present at this locus (98). In 1994, Kamb et al. published a study demonstrating that the 9p21 locus, previously implicated in melanoma oncogenesis, contains p16, and this gene is mutated in melanoma cell lines (99). Recent studies have demonstrated that mutated tumor-derived alleles of p16 found in melanomas are deficient in blocking the GI/S phase transition of the cell cycle because of ineffective inhibition of cyclin-dependent kinase 4 (100,101).

The INK4a locus produces two transcripts, one of which encodes p16, designated E1α; the other transcript (E1b) has recently been shown to encode a 19 kilodalton molecule in an alternative reading frame (102). Both p16 and p19 appear to regulate cell cycle progression (102,103); it will be interesting to see how base mutations at this shared locus influence p16 and p19 function and the evolution of melanocytic neoplasia. Other potential candidate genes involved in melanomagenesis may exist on chromosomes 1, 6, 7, 10 and 11 (104). Further investigation of p16 and p19 signaling pathways and other chromosomal loci will provide additional insights into the evolution of melanocytic oncogenesis.

V. SUMMARY

Nevi and Dysplastic Nevi are Risk Markers, Potential Precursors, and Simulants of Melanoma

The data reviewed above are consistent with a model of tumor progression in which melanomas evolve from cutaneous melanocytes through a series of nonobligatory lesional steps, any of which can be bypassed ("telescoped" tumor progression). In the first of these steps, melanocytes may acquire mutations of DNA induced by ultraviolet light, resulting in the formation of benign tumors (nevi). There may be variations in individual susceptibility related to poorly understood age-related factors and to genetic defects in protective factors such as pigmentary characteristics and DNA repair mechanisms. Particular melanocytic nevi may be more susceptible than others to continuing injury because of poor shielding of lesional melanocytes from UVB and because of abnormal pheomelanin pigment that generates toxic free radicals on exposure to light. The continuing action of ultraviolet light may drive an increasingly unstable tumor progression system, with increasing atypia leading first to changes of clinical atypia and histologic dysplasia and then to other attributes of the malignant phenotype such as invasion and tumorigenic proliferation. Ultraviolet light may also contribute to tumor progression by its immunosuppressive effect (105). In this model, nevi, especially dysplastic nevi, occupy a pivotal position as risk markers, potential precursors, and simulants of melanoma, similar to dysplastic lesions in other tumor systems.

ACKNOWLEDGMENT

Supported by research grants CA-25298 and CA-25874 from the National Cancer Institute.

REFERENCES

1. Rous P, Beard JW. The progression to carcinoma of virus-induced papillomas (Shope). J Exp Med 1935; 62:523.
2. Foulds L. Neoplastic development. London and New York: Academic Press, 1969; 41–86.
3. Clark WH. Tumour progression and the nature of cancer. Br J Cancer 1991; 64:631.
4. Elder DE, Murphy GF. Malignant tumors (melanomas and related lesions). In: Elder DE, Murphy GF eds. Melanocytic tumors of the skin. Washington, D.C: Armed Forces Institute of Pathology, 1991; p 103.
5. Moolgavkar SH. Carcinogenesis models: An overview. Basic Life Sci 1991; 58:387.
6. Cook PJ, Doll R, Fellingham SA. A mathematical model for the age distribution of cancer in man. Int J Cancer 1969; 4:93.
7. Peto R, Roe FJ, Lee PN, Levy L, Clack J. Cancer and ageing in mice and men. Br J Cancer 1975; 32:411.
8. Den Otter W, Koten JW, Van der Vegt BJ, Beemer FA, Boxma OJ, Derkinderen DJ, De Graaf PW, Huber J, Lips CJ, Roholl PJ, et al. Oncogenesis by mutations in anti-oncogenes: A view. Anticancer Res 1990; 10:475.
9. Moolgavkar SH, Knudson AG. Mutation and cancer: A model for human carcinogenesis. JNCI 1981; 66:1037.
10. Fearon ER, Vogelstein B. A genetic model for colorectal carcinogenesis. Cell 1990; 61:759.
11. Whimster IW. Recurrent pigment cell naevi and their significance in the problem of endogenous carcinogenesis. Ann Ital Dermatol Clin Sper 1965; 19:168.
12. Hu F. Melanocyte cytology in normal skin, melanocytic nevi, and malignant melanomas. In: Ackerman AB, ed. Pathology of Malignant Melanoma. Masson, New York, 1981: 1.
13. Gallagher RP, McLean DI, Yang CP, Coldman AJ, Silver HKB, Spinelli JJ, Beagrie M. Suntan, sunburn, and pigmentation factors and the frequency of acquired melanocytic nevi in children: Similarities to melanoma: The Vancouver mole study. Arch Dermatol 1990; 126:770.
14. Halpern AC, Guerry DIV, Elder DE, Clark WH, Jr., Synnestvedt M, Norman S, Ayerle R: Dysplastic nevi as risk

markers of sporadic (non-familial) melanoma: A case-control study. Arch Dermatol 1991; 127:995.

15. Goovaerts G, Buyssens N. Nevus cell maturation or atrophy. Am J Dermatopathol 1988; 10:20.

16. Lund HZ, Stobbe GD. The natural history of the pigmented nevus: Factors of age and anatomic location. Am J Pathol 1949; 6:1117.

17. Wayte DM, Helwig EB. Halo nevi. Cancer 1968; 22:69.

18. Clark WH, Jr., Elder DE, Guerry DIV, Epstein MN, Greene MH, Van Horn M. A study of tumor progression: The precursor lesions of superficial spreading and nodular melanoma. Hum Pathol 1984; 15:1147.

19. Enomoto K, Farber E. Kinetics of phenotypic maturation or remodelling of hyperplastic nodules during liver carcinogenesis. Cancer Res 1982; 42:2330.

20. Feinberg SM, Jagelman DG, Sarre RG, McGannon E, Fazio VW, Lavery IC, Weakly FL, Easley KA. Spontaneous resolution of rectal polyps in patients with familial polyposis following abdominal colectomy and ileorectal anastomosis. Dis Colon Rect 1988; 31:169.

21. Holman CD, Armstrong BK. Pigmentary traits, ethnic origin, benign nevi, and family history as risk factors for cutaneous malignant melanoma. J Natl Cancer Inst 1984; 72:257.

22. Easton DF, Cox GM, Macdonald AM, Ponder BAJ. Genetic susceptibility to naevi—A twin study. Br J Cancer 1991; 64:1164.

23. Elder DE, Greene MH, Bondi EE, Clark WH, Jr. Acquired melanocytic nevi and melanoma: the dysplastic nevus syndrome. In: Ackerman, AB, ed. Pathology of malignant melanoma. New York, Masson, 1981: 185.

24. Holly EA, Kelly JW, Shpall SN, Chiu S-H. Number of melanocytic nevi as a risk factor for malignant melanoma. J Am Acad Dermatol 1987; 17:459.

25. Clark WH Jr, Reimer RR, Greene MH, Ainsworth AA, Mastrangelo MJ. Origin of familial melanomas from heritable melanocytic lesions. Arch Dermatol 1978; 114:732.

26. Reimer RR, Clark WH Jr, Greene MH, Ainsworth AM, Fraumeni JF, Jr. Precursor lesions in familial melanoma. A new genetic preneoplastic syndrome. JAMA 1978; 239:744.

27. Lynch HT, Frichot BCIIl. Lynch JF. Familial atypical multiple mole-melanoma syndrome. J Med Gene 1978; 15:352.

28. Greene MH, Clark WH Jr, Tucker MA, Elder DE, Kraemer KH, Fraser MC, Bondi EE, Guerry DIV, Tuthill R, Hamilton R, LaRossa D. Precursor naevi in cutaneous malignant melanoma: a proposed nomenclature [letter]. Lancet 1980; 2:1024.

29. Elder DE, Goldman LI, Goldman SC, Greene MH, Clark WH, Jr. Dysplastic nevus syndrome: a phenotypic association of sporadic cutaneous melanoma. Cancer 1980; 46:1787.

30. Osterlind A, Tucker MA, Stone BJ, Jensen OM. The Danish case-control study of cutaneous malignant melanoma. II. Importance of UV-light exposure. Int J Cancer 1988; 42:319.

31. Nordlund JJ, Kirkwood J, Forget BM, Scheibner A, Albert DM, Lerner E, Milton GW. Demographic study of clinically atypical (dysplastic) nevi in patients with melanoma and comparison subjects. Cancer Res 1985; 45:1855.

32. MacKie RM, Freudenberger T, Aitchison TC. Personal risk-factor chart for cutaneous melanoma. Lancet 1989; 2:487.

33. Augustsson A, Stierner U, Rosdahl I, Suurkula M. Sun exposure, common and dysplastic nevi in melanoma patients and controls. Abstracts, 2nd International Conference on Melanoma 34, 1989.

34. Garbe C, Kruger S, Stadler R, Guggenmoos-Holzmann I, Orfanos CE: Markers and relative risk in a German population for developing malignant melanoma. Int J Dermatol 1989; 28:517.

35. Kraemer KH, Greene MH, Tarone R, Elder DE, Clark WHJr, Guerry DIV. Dysplastic naevi and cutaneous melanoma risk [letter]. Lancet 1983; 2:1076.

36. National Institutes of Health. Precursors to malignant melanoma. National Institutes of Health, Oct 24–26, 1983. Am J Dermatopathol 1984; 6 Suppl:169.

37. Bergman W, Watson P, De Jong J, Lynch HT, Fusaro RM. Systemic cancer and the FAMMM syndrome. Br J Cancer 1990; 61:932.

38. Lynch HT, Fusaro RM. The surgeon, genetics, and malignant melanoma. Arch Surg 1992; 127:317.

39. Grob JJ, Andrac L, Romano MH, Davin D, Collet Villette AM, Munoz MH, Bonerandi JJ. Dysplastic naevus in non-familial melanoma. A clinicopathological study of 101 cases. Br J Dermatol 1988; 118:745.

40. Kopf AW, Friedman RJ, Rigel DS. Atypical mole syndrome. J Am Acad Dermatol 1990; 22:117.

41. Elder DE, Green MH, Guerry DIV, Kraemer KH, Clark WH, Jr. The dysplastic nevus syndrome: our definition. Am J Dermatopathol 1982; 4:455.

42. Greene MH, Clark WH, Jr., Tucker MA, Elder DE, Kraemer KH, Guerry DIV, Witmer WK, Thompson J, Matozzo I, Fraser MC. Acquired precursors of cutaneous malignant melanoma. The familial dysplastic nevus syndrome. N Engl J Med 1985; 312:91.

43. Friedman RJ, Heilman ER, Rigel DS, Kopf AW. The dysplastic nevus. Clinical and pathologic features. Dermatol Clin 1985; 3:239.

44. Elder DE, Murphy GF. Benign melanocytic tumors (nevi). In: Elder DE, Murphy GF, eds. Melanocytic tumors of the skin. Washington, D.C.: Armed Forces Institute of Pathology, 1991: 5.

45. Yamada K, Salopek T, Jimbow K, Ito S. An extremely high content of pheomelanin in dysplastic nevi. J Invest Dermatol 1989; 92:544a.

46. Kraemer KH, Greene MH, Tarone R. Dysplastic nevi and cutaneous melanoma risk. Letter. N Engl J Med 1987; 315:1615.

47. Greene M, Clark WHJr, Tucker MA, Kraemer KH, Elder DE, Fraser MC. High risk of malignant melanoma in melanoma-prone families with dysplastic nevi. Ann Intern Med 1985; 102:458.

48. Masri GD, Clark WHJr, Guerry DIV, Halpern A, Thompson CJ, Elder DE. Screening and surveillance of patients at high risk for malignant melanoma result in detection of earlier disease. J Am Acad Dermatol 1990; 22:1042.

49. Rhodes AR, Harrist TJ, Day CL, Mihm MC Jr, Fitzpatrick TB, Sober AJ. Dysplastic melanocytic nevi in histologic association with 234 primary cutaneous melanomas. J Am Acad Dermatol 1983; 9:563.

50. Cook MG, Robertson I. Melanocytic dysplasia and melanoma. Histopathology 1985; 9:647.
51. Maize JC, Ackerman AB. Pigmented lesions of the skin. Clinicopathologic correlations. Philadelphia: Lea & Febiger, 1987.
52. English DR, Menz J, Heenan PJ, Elder DE, Watt JD, Armstrong BK. The dysplastic naevus syndrome in patients with cutaneous malignant melanoma in Western Australia. Med J Aust 1986; 145:194.
53. Black WC. Residual dysplastic and other nevi in superficial spreading melanoma. Clinical correlations and association with sun damage. Cancer 1988; 62:163.
54. Hastrup N, Osterlind A, Drzewiecki KT, Hou-Jensen K: The presence of dysplastic nevus remnants in malignant melanomas: A population-based study of 551 malignant melanomas. Am J Dermatopathol 1991; 13:378.
55. Gruber SB, Barnhill RL, Stenn KS, Roush GC. Nevomelanocytic proliferations in association with cutaneous malignant melanoma: A multivariate analysis. J Am Acad Dermatol 1989; 21:773.
56. Clark WH, Jr., Elder DE, Guerry DIV. The pathogenesis and pathology of dysplastic nevi and malignant melanoma. In: Farmer E, Hood A, eds. The pathology of the skin. edited by New York: Appleton-Century-Crofts, 1989.
57. Elder DE, Murphy GF. Melanocytic tumors of the skin, Washington, D.C.: Armed Forces Institute of Pathology, 1991.
58. Halpern AC, Guerry D, Elder DE, Trock B, Synnestvedt M. A cohort study of melanoma in patients with dysplastic nevi. J Invest Dermatol 1993; 100:346S.
59. Piepkorn MW, Barnhill RL, Cannon-Albright LA, Elder DE, Goldgar DE, Lewis CM, Maize JC, Meyer LJ, Rabkin MS, Sagebiel RW, Skolnick MH, Zone JJ. A multi-observer, population-based analysis of histologic dysplasia in melanocytic nevi. (Submitted 1992.)
60. Augustsson A, Stierner U, Rosdahl I, Suurküla M. Common and dysplastic naevi as risk factors for cutaneous malignant melanoma in a Swedish population. Acta Derm Venereol (Stockh) 1991; 71:518.
61. Grob JJ, Gouvernet J, Aymar D, Mostaque A, Romano MH, Collet AM, Noe MC, Diconstanzo MP, Bonerandi JJ. Count of

benign melanocytic nevi as a major risk factor for nonfamilial nodular and superficial spreading melanoma. Cancer 1990; 66:387.

62. Meyer LJ, Goldgar DE, Cannon-Albright LA, Piepkorn MW, Zone JJ, Risman MB, Skolnick MH. Number, size, and histopathology of nevi in Utah kindreds. Cytogenet Cell Genet 1992; 59:167.

63. Goldgar DE, Cannon-Albright LA, Meyer LJ, Piepkorn MW, Zone JJ, Skolnick MH. Inheritance of nevus number and size in melanoma/DNS kindreds. Cytogenet Cell Gene 1992; 59:200.

64. Green A, Siskind V, Bain C, Alexander J. Sunburn and malignant melanoma. Br J Cancer 1985; 51:393.

65. Swerdlow AJ, English J, MacKie RM, O'Doherty CJ, Hunter JAA, Clark J, Hole DJ. Benign melanocytic naevi as a risk factor for malignant melanoma. Brit Med J 1986; 292:1555.

66. Roush GC, Nordlund JJ, Forget B, Gruber SB, Kirkwood JM. Independence of dysplastic nevi from total nevi in determining risk for nonfamilial melanoma. Prev Med 1988; 17:273.

67. Bale SJ, Chakravarti A, Greene MH: Cutaneous malignant melanoma: evidence for autosomal dominant inheritance and pleiotrophy. Am J Hum Genet 1986; 38:188.

68. Tucker MA, Fraser MC, Goldstein AM, Elder DE, Guerry DIV, Organic SM. The risk of melanoma and other cancers in melanoma-prone families. J Invest Dermatol 1992 (in press).

69. Carey WP, Jr., Thompson CJ, Synnestvedt M, Guerry D, Halpern A, Schultz D, Elder DE: Dysplastic nevi as a melanoma risk factor in patients with familial melanoma. Cancer 1994; 74:3118.

70. Rigel DS, Rivers JK, Kopf AW, Friedman RJ, Vinokur AF, Heilman ER, Levenstein M. Dysplastic nevi: Markers of increased risk for melanoma. Cancer 1989; 63:386.

71. Dabski K, Milgrom H, Stoll HL, Jr. Dysplastic nevus syndrome: Association with multiple primary neoplasms. J Surg Oncol 1986; 32:113.

72. Pehamberger H, Honigsmann H, Wolff K. Dysplastic nevus syndrome with multiple primary amelanotic melanomas in oculocutaneous albinism. J Am Acad Dermatol 1984; 11:731.

73. Sigg C, Pelloni F, Schnyder UW: Increased incidence of multiple melanoma in sporadic and familial dysplastic nevus syndrome. Hautarzt 1989; 40:548.
74. Titus Ernstoff L, Duray PH, Ernstoff MS, Barnhill RL, Horn PL, Kirkwood JM. Dysplastic nevi in association with multiple primary melanoma. Cancer Res 1988; 48:1016.
75. MacKie RM. Multiple melanoma and atypical melanocytic nevi—evidence of an activated and expanded melanocytic system. Br J Dermatol 1982; 107:621.
76. Jones PA, Buckley JD. The role of DNA methylation in cancer. Adv Cancer Res 1990; 54:1.
77. Elder DE, Rodeck U, Thurin J, Cardillo F, Clark WH, Jr., Stewart R, Herlyn M. Antigenic profile of tumor progression stages in human melanocytic nevi and melanomas. Cancer Res 1989; 49:5091.
78. Ruiter DJ, Dingjan GM, Steijlen PM, van Beveren Hooyer M, de Graaff ReitsmaC, Bergman W, van Muijen GN, Warnaar SO. Monoclonal antibodies selected to discriminate between malignant melanomas and nevocellular nevi. J Invest Dermatol 1985; 85:4.
79. van Muijen GN, Ruiter DJ, Hoefakker S, Johnson JP. Monoclonal antibody PAL-M1 recognizes the transferrin receptor and is a progression marker in melanocytic lesions. J Invest Dermatol 1990; 95:65.
80. Maeda K, Jimbow K. Positive reactivity of dysplastic melanocytes with a monoclonal antibody against melanoma melanosomes, MoAb HMSA-2. J Invest Dermatol 1988; 91:247.
81. Takahashi H, Parsons PG, Favier D, McEwan M, Strutton GM, Akutsu Y, Jimbow K. Complementary expression of melanosomal antigens and constant expression of pigment-independent antigen during the evolution of melanocytic tumours. Virchows Arch [A] 1990; 416:513.
82. Salopek TG, Yamada K, Ito S, Jimbow K. Dysplastic melanocytic nevi contain high levels of pheomelanin: quantitative comparison of pheomelanin/eumelanin levels between normal skin, common nevi, dysplastic nevi. Pigment Cell Res 1992 (in press).

83. Land EJ, Thomson A, Truscott TG, Subaro KV, Chedekel MR. Photochemistry of melanin precursors: Dopa, 5-S-cysteinyldopa and 2,5-S,S-cysteinyldopa. Photochem Photobiol 1986; 44:697.

84. Harsanyi ZP, Post PW, Brinkmann JP, Chedekel MR, Deibel RM. Mutagenicity of melanin from human red hair. Experiential 1980; 36:291.

85. Parmiter AH, Nowell PC. The cytogenetics of human melanoma and premalignant lesions. In: Nathanson L, ed. Malignant melanoma: Biology, diagnosis and therapy. Boston: Kluwer Academic Publishers, 1988:47.

86. Schmiegelow P, Schroiff R, Breitbart E, Bahnsen J, Lindner J, Janner M. Malignant melanoma—its precursors and topography of proliferation. Virchows Arch [Pathol Anat] 1986; 409:47.

87. Santucci M, Urso C, Giannini A, Bondi R. Common acquired melanocytic nevi, melanocytic dysplasia and malignant melanoma: A morphometric study. Appl Pathol 1989; 7:111.

88. Smith PJ, Greene MH, Devlin DA, McKeen EA, Paterson MC. Abnormal sensitivity to UV-radiation in cultured skin fibroblasts from patients with hereditary cutaneous malignant melanoma and dysplastic nevus syndrome. Int J Cancer 1982; 30:39.

89. Jung EG, Bohnert E, Boonen H. Dysplastic nevus syndrome: Ultraviolet hypermutability confirmed in vitro by elevated sister chromatid exchanges. Dermatological 1986; 173:297.

90. Jaspers NG, Roza de JonghEJ, Donselaar IG, Van Velzen Tillemans JT, van Hemel JO, Rumke P, van der Kamp AW. Sister chromatid exchanges, hyperdiploidy and chromosomal rearrangements studied in cells from melanoma-prone individuals belonging to families with the dysplastic nevus syndrome. Cancer Genet Cytogenet 1987; 24:33.

91. Perera MI, Um KI, Greene MH, Waters HL, Bredberg A, Kraemer KH. Hereditary dysplastic nevus syndrome: lymphoid cell ultraviolet hypermutability in association with increased melanoma susceptibility. Cancer Res 1986; 46:1005.

92. Roth M, Boyle JM, Muller H. Thymine dimer repair in fibrob-

lasts of patients with dysplastic naevus syndrome (DNS). Experientia 1988; 44:169.

93. Sanford KK, Tarone RE, Parshad R, Tucker MA, Greene MH, Jones GM. Hypersensitivity to G2 chromatid radiation damage in familial dysplastic naevus syndrome. Lancet 1987; 2:1111.

94. Hürlimann AF, Bohnert E, Schnyder UW, Jung EG. Dysplastic nevus syndrome: Intrafamilial identification of carriers by cytogenetics. Dermatological 1992; 184:223.

95. Pollock PM, Yu F, Qiu L, Parsons PG, Hayward NK. Evidence for uv induction of *CDKN2* mutations in melanoma cell lines. Oncogene 1995; 11:663.

96. Caporaso N, Greene MH, Tsai S, Pickle LW, Mulvihill JJ. Cytogenetics in hereditary malignant melanoma and dysplastic nevus syndrome: Is dysplastic nevus syndrome a chromosome instability disorder? Cancer Genet Cytogenet 1987; 24:299.

97. Jung EG. Photocarcinogenesis in the skin. J Dermatol 1991; 18:1.

98. Fountain JW, Karayiorgou M, Ernstoff MS, Kirkwood JM, Vlock DR, Titus-Ernstoff L, Bouchard B, Vijayasaradhi S, Houghton AN, Lahti J, Kidd VJ, Housman DE, Dracopoli NC. Homozygous deletions within human chromosome band 9p21 in melanoma. Proc Natl Acad Sci USA 1992; 89:10557.

99. Kamb A, Gruis NA, Weaver-Feldhaus J, Liu Q, Harshman K, Tavtigian SV, Stockert E, Day R.S III, Johnson BE, Skolnick M. A cell cycle regulator potentially involved in genesis of many tumor types. Science 1994; 264:436.

100. Reymond A, Brent R. p16 proteins from melanoma-prone families are deficient in binding to Cdk4. Oncogene 1995; 11:1173.

101. Koh J, Enders GH, Dynlacht BD, Harlow E. Tumor-derived p16 alleles encoding proteins defective in cell-cycle regulation. Nature 1995; 375:507.

102. Quelle DE, Zindy F, Ashmun RA, Sherr CJ. Alternative reading frames of the INK4a tumor suppressor gene encodes two unrelated proteins capable of inducing cell cycle arrest. Cell 1995; 83:993.

103. Serrano M, Hannon GJ, Beach D. A new regulatory motif in cell cycle control causing specific inhibition of cyclinD/cdk4. Nature 1993; 366:704.
104. Trent JM. Cytogenetics of human malignant melanoma. Cancer Metastasis Rev 1991; 10:103.
105. Cruz PD, Jr., Bergstresser PR. Ultraviolet radiation, Langerhans' cells, and skin cancer: Conspiracy and failure. Arch Dermatol 1989; 125:975.

Part III
Adjuvant Therapy of Resected Cutaneous High-Risk Melanoma

4

LYMPHATIC MAPPING AND SENTINEL LYMPH NODE BIOPSY IN THE CARE OF THE PATIENT WITH MELANOMA

Douglas S. Reintgen and Andrea Brobeil

Moffitt Cancer Center and Research Institute
University of South Florida
Tampa, Florida

I. INTRODUCTION

In the surgical management of cutaneous melanoma, many physicians have been presented with the dilemma of performing an elective lymph node dissection (ELND) or of following the "wait and watch" method of observing the regional basin. Opponents of ELND cite the morbidity associated with the procedure and prefer instead to follow patients closely, and to perform a therapeutic lymph node dissection (TLND) only of nodal disease becomes clinically apparent. This strategy spares patients without nodal involvement the morbidity associated with a complete lymph node dissection (CLND) (1). Proponents of ELND, however, argue that the treatment is effective because it removes micrometastases which, if left untreated may act as the source of further nodal and perhaps systemic disease. The concern is that by the time the lymph node is clinically detected, disease may have already spread to higher-order nodes or to distant sides (1).

Although these two schools of thought differ in practice, both agree on the value of nodal status as a prognostic indicator, and both recognize the importance of removing involved nodes. Combined with preoperative lymphoscintigraphy and intraoperative lymphatic mapping, selective lymphadenectomy now offers a compromise between the traditional alternatives of either ELND or observation of the regional nodal basin.

II. THE SENTINEL LYMPH NODE

The sentinel lymph node (SLN) is defined as the first node in the lymphatic basin to which the primary melanoma drains (Fig. 1; see insert). Since the SLN is the node receiving primary lymphatic flow, it is also the node most likely to be positive for metastatic disease. If this SLN can be successfully identified and localized, it offers an accurate reflection of the histology of the rest of the basin (2). That is, if the SLN is negative, the remainder of the basin should also be negative; however, if the SLN is positive, additional or higher-order nodes may also be positive. This information can be used to direct surgical management of the patient, subjecting only node-positive patients to the expense and morbidity of a CLND (3).

III.   PREOPERATIVE LYMPHOSCINTIGRAPHY

The benefits of selective lymphadenectomy, or SLN biopsy, all stem from the surgeon's ability to identify the basin at risk for metastatic disease and the individual nodes in the basin most at risk. However, traditionally accepted patterns of lymphatic drainage have been proven in dynamic studies in patients to be too simplistic and are no longer used in making such predictions. In 1874, Sappey used mercury injections in cadavers to observe patterns of lymphatic flow in humans (4). He determined that humans had a line of demarcation running along the midline and from just above the umbilicus and curving backward toward the second lumbar vertebra. Lesions above "Sappey's line" were thought to drain to the ipsilateral axilla whereas lesions below the line drained to the ipsilateral groin; likewise, lesions to the left of the midline were thought to drain to the left axilla or groin and lesions to the right of the midline were thought to drain to the right axilla or groin. "Watershed" areas of bidirectional flow were proposed to exist 2.5 cm on each side of the midline and 2.5 cm on each side of Sappey's line. This "watershed" area was thought to be so small that it was considered inconsequential.

Norman and colleagues (5), however, found that there existed a much wider watershed area than Sappey had described (Fig. 2). They argued that, in actuality, a physician cannot accurately predict lymphatic drainage using traditional guidelines until the cutaneous lesion is 11 cm on either side of Sappey's line or the midline. The only areas of

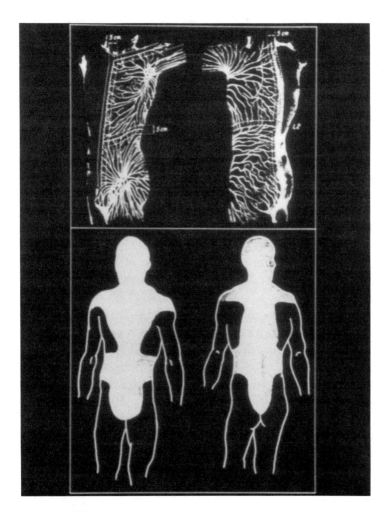

FIGURE 2 Diagram showing "watershed" areas of the body. Norman et al. (5) found the areas of ambiguous drainage to be larger than those reported by Sappey (4). (Top) Sappey's classic anatomical drainage patterns. (Bottom) Norman's map of multidirectional flow. Melanomas at primary sites depicted in the shaded area may have multidirectional flow, and preoperative lymphoscintigraphy is necessary.

anatomically predictable drainage are areas centered around the axilla, lateral hip, and extremity. In addition, a study from Moffitt Cancer Center (MCC) found that 33% of the time, the physician could not predict the location of the SLN within 5 cm. Preoperative lymphoscintigraphy, however, succeeded in accurately locating the SLN in the basin within 1 cm, 100% of the time (25).

The unpredictable nature of lymphatic drainage and this concept of multidirectional cutaneous flow have emphasized the need for a preoperative localizing study. Without one, the correct regional basin may not be located, much less the individual SLN. Preoperative lymphoscintigraphy is a nuclear medicine imaging study that identifies all regional basins at risk for metastasis as well as the node in the basin receiving primary lymphatic flow. The first node, or the SLN, is consequently at high risk for metastatic disease. Preoperative lymphoscintigraphy directly assists in planning the surgical procedure by: (1) identifying all nodes at risk for metastatic disease, (2) identifying any intransit nodes, defined as nodes between the primary site and the regional basin, (3) identifying the location of the SLN in relation to the rest of the nodes in the nodal basin, and (4) estimating the number of SLNs (14) (Fig. 3).

Preoperative lymphoscintigraphy involves the intradermal injection of approximately 450 µCi of filtered technetim-99m sulfur colloid (Medi-Physics, Inc. , Arlington Heights, IL) in four parts distributed circumferentially around the biopsy site. A large field-of-view gamma camera fitted with a low-energy, high-resolution parallel-hole collimator is used to image the patient. The body outline is obtained by placing a cobalt flood source between the patient and the camera for 30 sec. Images are obtained in the head, neck, chest, abdomen, and pelvis. One hundred thousand counts are obtained for anterior-posterior and lateral views and are recorded on film. After scans of the primary site are made immediately on injection, a dynamic flow study is obtained to identify the SLN. With early 10-min. scans, an afferent lymphatic is usually identified leading to the SLN. With early 10-min. scans, an afferent lymphatic is usually identified leading to the SLN, and the location of the SLN is marked with an intradermal tattoo. Delayed 2-hr. images are taken to ensure no late drainage to another basin, and the presence of tracer in the liver is documented to verify ymphatic uptake.

After viewing the patient's preoperative lymphoscintigrams, the surgeon is better equipped to perform the SLN biopsy. The radiocolloid, technetium-sulfur colloid has the correct particle size to be taken up in the lymphatic channels in much the same way that metastatic cells travel from the primary site to the regional basin. The surgeon now knows the most likely routes for metastatic disease and the most likely node in the basin to harbor these metastatic cells.

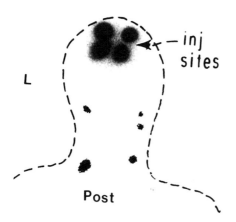

FIGURE 3 Lymphoscintigram showing the posterior view of a patient with head-and-neck melanoma. The patient was injected around the primary-site scar with technetium-99m sulfur colloid and bilateral posterior chain drainage was identified. Both basins are equally at risk for metastatic disease, and both basins should have SLNs identified.

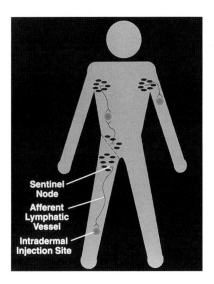

FIGURE 1 Schematic of the SLN concept. Primary injection site and the afferent lymphatic leading to the SLN. Lymphatic mapping using technetium-99m sulfur colloid and blue dye (featured here) assists the surgeon in identifying the SLN. Both agents are taken up by the cutaneous lymphatics and deposited in the SLN. The SLN, or node(s) most at risk for metastatic disease, will be identified as either "hot" with radioactivity or blue-stained with vital blue dye. Primary melanomas that drain in multiple directions can be mapped and the SLN(s) identified in each basin.

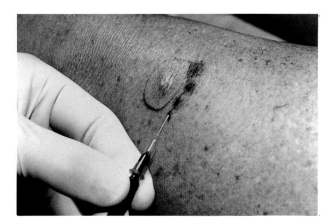

FIGURE 4 Injection of isosulfan blue. The vital blue dye is injected intradermally and circumferentially around the biopsy site to create a wheal. The dye travels through the afferent lymphatics, as would metastatic cells, and will color the first node blue, giving the surgeon a visual clue as to where the SLN is located.

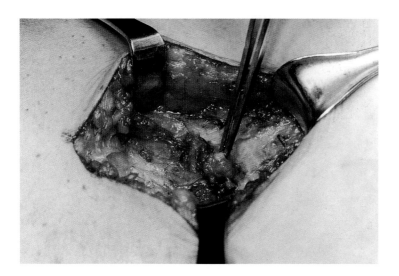

FIGURE 5 Intraoperative mapping. The surgeon identifies two blue-stained afferent lymphatics converging to the SLN (forceps) in the groin of a patient with an intermediate thickness melanoma from the calf.

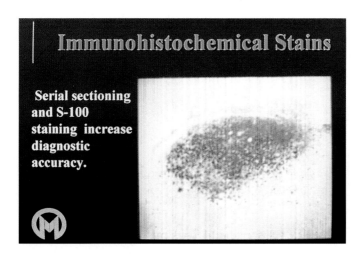

FIGURE 6 S-100 immunohistochemical stain showing a deposit of micrometastatic melanoma in the SLN of a patient with an inter-mediate-thickness melanoma. The metastatic cells stain brown while the normal lymphocytes in the node do not stain. Compared to standard histological examination, immunohistochemical staining can improve sensitivity of the occult metastasis assay by a factor of 10, being able to identify one abnormal melanoma cell in a background of 10^5 lymphocytes.

Armed with this road map of potential lymphatic spread, the surgeon can design his operation to remove or sample only and all those nodal basins at risk for disease.

IV. INTRAOPERATIVE LYMPHATIC MAPPING

After the preoperative lymphoscintigraphy has identified the correct nodal basin(s) at risk for metastatic disease and the node in the basin most at risk, the surgeon must then locate the node in vivo.

Intraoperative lymphatic mapping and SLN biopsy was initially proposed by Morton el al. (7) who described a vital blue dye mapping technique. Protocols established at MCC use a combination of vital blue dye and radiolymphoscintigraphy to assist the surgeon intraoperatively, to increase the success rate of SLN localization and to decrease the steep learing curve.

A. Vital Blue Dye

The intraoperative lymphatic mapping procedure involves the intradermal injection of Lymphazurine Blue (Zenity Parenterals, Rosemont, IL) around the biopsy site to create a wheel (Fig. 4; see insert). One milliliter of dye is used if the melanoma drains in 1 direction, and 2 ml are used if 2 nodal basins are at risk. Morton et al. found isosulfan blue to be the most effective dye, as it is taken up quickly by the lymphatic vessels with very little diffusion to the surrounding tissue (22). Side effects of isosulfan blue are minimal and include: (1) rare reports of allergic reactions, (2) presence of dye in the urine during the first 24 h, and (3) possible interference with transcutaneous oxygen monitoring during anesthesia (14). For the most part, however, there are few complications.

After the injection, a small incision is made at the tattoo marker, and the surgeon can follow the blue-stained afferent lymphatic, leading to the SLN (Fig. 5; see insert). This blue node is harvested and sent to pathology for histological examination Morton et al, reported successfully identifying 194 of 237 lymphatic basins and detecting metastasis in 40 specimens (21%) by routine histological examination (1). Forty-seven of 259 SLNs (18%) were positive for metastatic disease but only 1 of 3079 non-SLNs were found to be positive in CLND specimens. This yields a false negative rate of less than 1%. With a success rate of 82% in SLN identification of his initial 170 patients, Morton's group finds blue dye mapping to be an accurate method of identifying the SLN.

The vital blue dye mapping technique made the SLN biopsy a viable procedure by facilitating the visual identification of the SLN. However, mapping using blue dye alone requires a considerable amount of experience and can result in an extensive dissection. Morton describes a learning curve of at least 60 cases to master this technique. It is not uncommon for community surgeons to see less than 60 melanoma cases in their lifetimes. One must question the widespread applicability of a technique when the learing curve is so steep (7.22).

In response to the shortcomings of blue dye mapping, intraoperative radiolymphoscintigraphy was developed to offer an easier and more accurate method of locating the SLN. This procedure serves as an effective complement to the blue dye mapping technique.

B. Radiolymphoscintigraphy

Intraoperative use of the Neoprobe (Neoprobe Corporation, Dublin, OH), or hand-held gamma counter, increases the success rate and decreases the learning curve for surgeons when compared to the use of vital blue dye alone. Since the preoperative lymphoscintigraphy is imaged the day before surgery, 450 µCi of technetium-99m sulfur colloid is reinjected around the biopsy site. After prepping and draping the patient, the surgeon uses the probe to examine the tattoo (left from the preoperative lymphoscintigraphy), marking the location of the SLN in the lymphatic basin. A small incision is made over the basin so that the SLN can be incorporated into the incision for a complete node dissection. Once through the skin and subcutaneous fat, the probe is aimed multidirectionally and gamma counts are monitored. The surgeon uses the Neoprobe as a navigation tool by proceeding to areas that the probe identifies as "hot" (i.e. they have high gamma counts with respect to background). The counts are followed to the first SLN, and the vital blue dye acts as a visual clue to confirm the location of the SLN. If the in vivo counts meet or exceed 3:1 (SLN/background, the node is considered a SLN. This procedure continues until all nodes located on the preoperative lymphoscintigraphy have been identified.

V. COMBINED BLUE DYE MAPPING AND RADIOLYMPHOSCINTIGRAPHY

While blue dye provides a visual road map for the surgeon to follow, the nature of the dye itself often causes it to be less than 100% reliable. Because it travels rapidly through the lymphatics, it may not remain in the nodes long enough for surgical identification and excision (8). Brobeil et al. documented a case where two of three metastatic nodes were "hot" but not blue, and if not for the Neoprobe, disease in these two nodes would have been missed (9). Due to reliable migration of radiocolloid, a significant prognostic indicator (nodal status) was identified. And because the number of involved nodes has been shown to affect survival (10,11), the probe contributed significantly to this patient's prognosis and management.

Combination intraoperative mapping was first performed at MCC and will provide the easiest method and highest success rate for finding the SLN(s). The vital blue dye and radiocolloid are complementary. Additionally, the Neoprobe's ability to examine the lymphatic basin through the skin lessens the need for extensive flaps and dissections. Blue dye alone may make the initial incision less precise. Another advantage of the radiocolloid mapping technique is that the surgeon may have a directed dissection through the basin to the level of nodes. For instance, in the axilla, a surgeon may have 5–10 cm of fat to dissect through until the level of nodes is reached. It can be tedious and frustrating for the surgeon to try to follow a "wisp" of blue-stained afferent lymphatics through 10 cm of fat. With the Neoprobe, the dissection is directed and minimized. The last advantage of radiocolloid mapping is that after the first SLN is removed, the basin can be scanned and, if all the SLNs have been removed, the radioactivity in the basin should return to background. If it does not, then the surgeon realizes he may have a second and third SLN in the basin that are equally at risk for metastatic disease. The mean number of SLNs removed in the melanoma population is 1.8 SLNs per patient, and more often than not, there is more than just a single SLN. If the surgeon were relying on just the vital blue dye to find the SLN, he would have to do an extensive dissection in the axilla, groin, or head and neck area to assure that all the blue-stained nodes have been removed from the basin. With the Neoprobe, one can simply scan the basin. With these advantages, the SLN biopsy is ideally a minimally invasive procedure, which 25% of the time allows for local anesthesia in an outpatient setting (particularly with groin dissections), thus sparing the patient additional expense.

This is not to say, however, that blue dye lymphography is not useful. In primary sites in close proximity to the regional lymph node basin, blue dye becomes a crucial part of the mapping procedure. Primary sites near regional basins are difficult to map due to radioactive "shine through" from the injection site. In these cases, the high gamma counts are actually emitted from the primary tumor site, rather than the SLN, and background counts are high. Blue dye provides a visual guide in these cases when radioactive counts may give ambiguous mapping directions.

Blue dye mapping and radiolymphoscintigraphy complement each other in guiding the surgeon to the SLNs. In a study performed at MCC, 70% of the SLNs demonstrated blue dye staining and 84% of the SLNs were considered "hot" (24). With a combined sensitivity of 96%, there is not a good reason to not use a combination mapping technique. Opponents of radiolymphoscintigraphy often cite its cost as a deterrent. However, after a cost analysis of technology associated with the lymphatic mapping procedure was performed, lymphatic mapping used for obtaining nodal staging information was found to be a cost-effective procedure (13). For the 38,300 new cases of melanoma diagnosed each year in the United States, obtaining nodal staging information with this new technology (as opposed to performing ELND) results in substantial projected savings for the health care industry. This group documents less patient morbidity, more accurate nodal staging, and an earlier return to work. Considering these long-term savings, the initial investment in technology seems minimal.

VI. REVERSE TRANSCRIPTASE-POLYMERASE CHAIN REACTION (RT-PCR)

At MCC only those patients with a positive SLN are subjected to a CLND. In an early study, 22% of the patients with a positive SLN had further metastatic disease, supporting the idea that patients with a positive SLN should have a CLND. A later MCC study showed this figure to drop to 6% when lymphatic mapping is performed for earlier-stage patients. Data from M.D. Anderson Cancer Center and MCC have been compiled on 423 patients who underwent lymphatic mapping and had a negative SLN biopsy. Twelve of these patients have recurred in their regional basins, and a detailed examination of the SLN in these patients (i.e. serial sectioning, immunohistochemical staining, and RT-PCR analysis) found some evidence for metastatic disease in 83%. The implication is that these false negative SLN biopsies do not represent a failed surgical mapping, but rather the inadequacies of routine histological examination.

The limitations of current pathological examinations have led to attempts to establish more sensitive assays for occult metastasis based on reverse transcriptase-polymerase chain reaction (RT-PCR). Approximately 25% of all patients with stage I and II melanoma (no nodal involvement) will recur and die of disease within 5 years of diagnosis. Some of these patients may have had hematogenous spread, rather than lymphatic spread, but a significant portion of them may have had missed regional draining lymph nodal micrometastases (14).

The standard histopathology interpretation using hematoxylin-eosin (H&E) staining is sensitive to the order of finding 1 abnormal cell in a background of 10^4 normal cells. However, the routine examination, cutting one to two sections of the central cross-section and staining with H&E, studies only 1–5% of the submitted material. With the addition of immunohistochemical staining with S-100 or HMB-45, sensitivity is improved to finding 1 melanoma cell in a background of 10^5 lymphocytes (Fig. 6; see insert) (15,16). When used together, serial sectioning and immunohistochemical staining have been proven to improve sensitivity and to increase yield of occult metastases.

Smith et al. in 1991 reported using RT-PCR to detect melanoma cells in the peripheral blood. By detecting the messenger RNA of tyrosinase, a key enzyme involved during the synthesis of melanin (17,18) one can be fairly certain that micrometastases are also present in the sample. Because melanocytes are not found under normal conditions in the lymph nodes or peripheral blood, the presence of mRNA-tyrosinase-positive cells indicates the presence of melanin-producing cells and thus micrometastatic disease.

In an initial study from MCC, Wang and colleagues documented 11 of 29 lymph nodes from 29 patients with intermediate-thickness melanomas to be pathologically positive (19). However, an additional 8 lymph nodes were found to be positive using RT-PCR. All nodes that were pathologically positive were also RT-PCR positive, showing the improved sensitivity of standard histopathological examination. An updated report from the same institution (26) cites a 60.9% recurrence rate among 23 patients both histologically and PCR positive (14/23). And among those who were both histologically and PCR negative, only 2.3% (1/44) recurred. The one patient who recurred had a local recurrence, and one can argue that these metastatic cells had not yet migrated to the regional basin at the time of the SLN harvest. As in the previous study, there were no specimens that were PCR negative but histologically positive.

The relevance of this increased number of positive nodes lies in the prospect of more accurate staging. In another study performed at MCC, 47% of the pathologically node-negative patients were upstaged to stage III with RT-PCR (14). In this way RT-PCR can potentially identify patients who are likely to benefit from interferon alfa-2b, as determined by the Eastern Cooperative Oncology Group (ECOG) Trial 1684 (20) (see chapter 5). The benefit of the SLN biopsy and a more detailed pathological examination of the SLN is that it provides more accurate staging and has changed the standard of surgical care for patients with melanoma. Even those patients with melanomas greater than 4.0 mm in thickness can be offered SLN biopsy as a staging procedure since adjuvant Interferon alfa-2b seems to be most effective in the patient with nodal metastasis. Patients with thick melanomas and nodal involvement have a worse prognosis than patients with thick melanomas and no nodal involvement. Consequently, management for even this group can be better directed with a SLN biopsy.

VII. CONCLUSION

SLN biopsy offers a resolution to the dilemma posed by the previous options of ELND and observation. Because the histology of the SLN reflects the histology of the remainder of the lymphatic basin, only those patients with a positive SLN need undergo the morbidity of a CLND. The combined use of preoperative lymphoscintigraphy and intraoperative mapping with vital blue dye and radiolymphoscintigraphy results in a more accurate mapping with a minimally invasive procedure. In turn, a long-term reduction of costs for both the patient and the health care system is achieved. And with the use of RT-PCR, more micrometastases have been detected in SLNs, resulting in an "upstaging" for many patients with pathologically negative nodes. Such upstaging identifies patients who are most likely to benefit from adjuvant therapy.

Two prospective randomized trials, the Multicenter Selective Lymphadenectomy Trial (MSLT) and the Sunbelt Melanoma Trial (SMT), are currently investigating the efficacy of the lymphatic mapping and SLN biopsy procedures. The MSLT includes patients with Clark level III and Breslow thickness 1.00 mm or greater. The study randomizes these patients to either wide excision alone or wide excision combined with selective lymphadenectomy. If the SLN biopsy finds tumor-containing lymph nodes, a CLND is performed. The purpose of the study is to determine whether the SLN biopsy does, in fact, provide more accurate staging of melanoma and whether it better identifies patients who may benefit from a CLND. The study attempts to show a disease-free and overall survival benefit with the strategy of performing CLND only in those patients with proven micrometastatic disease, those with a positive SLN biopsy.

The ECOG 1684 trial included patients who generally (80% of the study population) had gross nodal disease, and data from this trial was the impetus for the FDA approval of Interferon alfa-2b as the first effective adjuvant theraphy for the high-risk-for-recurrence melanoma population. Patients with microscopic nodal disease only accounted for 9% of the ECOG 1684 population, and the effect of adjuvant therapy in the stage IIB population was not fully addressed because of the small number of patients in this subgroup.

In response to ECOG trial 1684, the Sunbelt Melanoma Trial will investigate the hypothesis that interferon alfa-2b has the greatest benefit for patients with early nodal metastatic disease. Patients with melanoma greater than 1.0 mm in thickness will undergo lymphatic mapping and SLN biopsy. Both the SLN and peripheral blood will be analyzed for markers of melanoma with the RT-PCR assay. If the SLN is histologically negative and PCR negative, the patient will be observed. If the SLN is histologically negative but PCR positive, the patient will be randomized to either observation, CLND, or CLND and Interferon alfa-2b. In this way, not only will the PCR assay's impact on prognosis be ascertained, but also the impact of treatment for the patient with a histologically negative, PCR-positive SLN will be examined. A second randomization will occur in patients who have only one histologically positive SLN. These patients will be randomized to receive either a CLND and observation or a CLND and interferon alfa-2b. This arm of the study will attempt to determine the role of adjuvant therapy in patients with microscopic disease. If the lymphatic mapping for this group yields more than 2 histologically positive SLNs, any positive non-SLNs, or any positive SLNs with gross extracapsular extension, the patient would not be randomized and would be offered standard adjuvant therapy.

The multidisciplinary nature of the SLN biopsy procedure requires close cooperation between surgeons, nuclear radiologists, and pathologists. Performing this technique without proper support is not in the best interest of the patient, as lower success rates in localization and inaccurate nodal staging may result. With the appropriate multidisciplinary team in place, lymphatic mapping, SLN biopsy, and a more detailed examination of the SLN may be anticipated to be more accurate in identifying micrometastases, providing a better prognostic assessment of patients with melanoma.

REFERENCES

1. Morton DL, Wen D-R, Wong JH, Economou JS, Cagie LA, Storm FK, et al. Technical details of intraoperative lymphatic mapping for early stage melanoma. Arch Surg 1992; 127:392–399.
2. Godellas CV, Berman CG, Lyman G, Cruse CW, Rapaport D, Heller R, et al. The identification and mapping of melanoma regional nodal metastasis: minimally invasive surgery for the diagnosis of nodal metastases. Am Surg 1995; 61:97–101.
3. Reintgen DS. Melanoma nodal metastases. Biologic significance and therapeutic considerations. Surg Clin North Am 1996; 5:105.
4. Sappey MPC. Anatomie, physiolgie, pathologie, des vaisscaux lymphatiques consideres chez les'homme et les vertegres. Paris: A DeLahaye and E Lecrosnier, 1874.
5. Norman J, Cruse CW, Espinos C, Cox C, Berman C, Clark R, et al. Redefinition of cutaneous lymphatic drainage with the use of lymphoscintigraphy for malignant melanoma. Am J Surg 1991; 162:432–437.
6. Berman CG, Norman J, Cruse CW, Reintgen DS, Clark RA. Lymphoscintigraphy in malignant melnoma. Ann Plast Surg 1992; 28:29–227.
7. Morton DL, Wen DR, Wong JH, et al. Technical details of intraoperative lymphatic mapping for early stage melanoma. Arch Surg 1992; 127–392.
8. Alazraki N. Lymphoscintigraphy and the intraoperative gamma probe. J Nucl Med 1995; 36:1780–1783.
9. Brobeil A, Kamath D, Cruse CW, Rapaport D, Well KE, Shons AR, et al. The clinical relevance of sentinel symph nodes identified with radiolymphoscintigraphy. J Flor Med Assoc 1997; 84:157–160.
10. Buzaid A, Tinoco L, Jendiroba D, et al. Prognostic value of

lymph node metastasis in patients with cutaneous melanoma. J CLin Oncol 1995; 13:2361–2368.

11. Balch C, Soong S-J, Shaw H, et al. Ananalysis of prognostic factors in 8500 patients with cutaneous melanoma. In: Balch C, Houghton A, Milton G, et al, eds. Cutaneous Melanoma 2nd ed. Philadelphia: JB Lippincott, 1992: 165–187.

12. Gershenwald J, Thompson W, Manfield P, et al. Patterns of failure in melanoma patients after successful lymphatic mapping and negative sentinel node biopsy. 49th Annual Cancer Symposium, Society of Surgical Oncology, Atlanta, GA, 1996 (abstract).

13. Reintgen DS, Albertini J, Miliotes G, Washburn J, Cruse CW, Rapaport D, et al. Investments in new technology research can save future health care dollars. J Flor Med.Assoc 1997; 84:175–181.

14. Reintgen DS, Rapaport DP, Tanabe KK, Ross MI. Lymphatic mapping and sentinel lymphadenectomy.

15. Cho KH, Hashimoto K, Taniguchi Y, et al. Immunohistochemical study of melanocytic nevus and malignant melanoma with monoclonal antibodies against S-100 subunits. Cancer 1990; 66:765–771.

16. Walts AE, Said JW, Shintaku IP. Cytodiagnosis of malignant melanoma: immunoperoxidase staining with HMB-45 antibody as an aid to diagnosis. Am J Clin Pathol 1988; 90:77–80.

17. Prota G. Recent advances in the chemistry of melanogenesis in mammals. J Invest Dermatol 1980; 75:122–127.

18. Slominski A, Constantino R. Molecular mechanism of tyrosinase regulastion by L-dopa in hamster melanoma cells. Life Sci 1987; 48:7473–7477.

19. Wang X, Heller R, VanNoorhis N, Cruse CW, Glass F, Fenske N, et al. Detection of submicroscopic lymph node metastases with polymerase chain reaction in patients with maligant melanoma.

20. Kirkwood JM, Strawderman MH, Ernstoff MS, et al. Adjuvant therapy of high-risk resected cutaneous melanoma. The Eastern Cooperative Oncology Group Trial EST 1684. J Clin Oncol 1996.

21. Wong JH, Cagle LA, Morton D. Lymphatic drainage of skin to

a sentinel lymph node in a feline model. Ann Surg 1991; 214:637.

22. Morton DL, Wen DR, Wong JH, et al. Technical details of intraoperative lymphatic mapping and selective lymphadenectomy or "watch and wait." Surg Oncol Clin North Am 1992; 1:247.

24. Albertini J, Cruse CW, Rapaport D, et al. Intraoperative radiolymphoscintigraphy improves sentinel lymph node identification in melnaoma patients. Ann Surg 1996; 223:217.

25. Miliotes G, Albertini J, Berman C, Heller R, Messina J, Glass F, et al. The tumor biology of melanoma nodal metastases. Am Surg 1996; 62:81–87.

26. Shivers S, Wang X, Li W, Rapaport D, Cruse CW, DeConti R, et al. Molecular staging of malignant melanoma—correlation with clinical outcome. N Engl J Med. Submitted.

5

MOLECULAR APPROACHES TO ADJUVANT IMMUNOLOGICAL THERAPY OF MELANOMA WITH INTERFERON (IFN)

The Role of Interferons and Other Cytokines as an Adjunct to Surgery in Intermediate- and High-Risk Melanoma

John M. Kirkwood

University of Pittsburgh School of Medicine and
University of Pittsburgh Cancer Institute
Pittsburgh, Pennsylvania

I. BACKGROUND

Melanoma incidence and mortality continue to rise around the world. Despite the recent substantial increase in our understanding of the molecular biology and immunology of this neoplasm, it has not yet been possible to demonstrate a reproducible significant impact of any systemic therapy upon the survival rate of patients with metastatic melanoma. A wide range of single agents and combinations of chemotherapeutic agents has been explored for the treatment of patients at high and intermediate risk of relapse, as reviewed elsewhere in this volume (see Bedikian and Legha, Chapter 8). The antihelminthic immunomodulator levamisole has shown improved survival in one study performed by the National Cancer Institute of Canada (NCIC) Melanoma Clinical Trials Group (1), but not in several other studies (2–4). Radiotherapy, which has palliative benefits for symptomatic metastatic disease, has also never been shown to alter relapse-free or overall survival in prospective randomized controlled trials. Newer techniques of stereotactic radiotherapy may have an impact in patients with a limited burden of metastatic disease, although this remains to be formally evaluated (see Flickinger et al., Chapter 10).

The first agent to prolong survival and interval to relapse in large multicenter, randomized, phase III trials is the pleiotropic biological agent interferon alfa2b (IFNα2b), as reported in the past year by the Eastern Cooperative Oncology Group (ECOG) Melanoma Committee (5). This chapter will present an overview and analysis of the results obtained with IFNα2b in the pivotal positive trial and place these results in the context of other past and current trials of the IFNs, and the literature of adjuvant systemic therapy of melanoma.

II. PROGNOSIS

A large number of factors have been evaluated for their importance in melanoma. In primary melanoma, the simple prognostic factors available to the clinician and investigator have recently been reviewed (6). In Chapter 4 of this volume, Reintgen and Brobeil have reviewed the sentinel lymph node mapping technique and the improved precision now available for surgical evaluation of lymphatic dissemination of cutaneous melanoma. Further, Keilholz and Willhauck (see Chapter 11) have summarized the literature and recent advances with potentially more sensitive and precise nested reverse transcriptase polymerase chain reaction (RT-PCR) measures of circulating tumor cell burden. The sentinel node mapping technique has already entered clinical practice, and molecular assays may, in the future, also become an element in decisions regarding whether or not to pursue adjuvant therapy and the assessment of clinical response in metastatic melanoma. For the present, the meaning of RT-PCR-defined regional lymph node and circulating tumor cell burden has yet to be established as a guide to the therapy of metastatic disease, for the selection and more precise definition of high-risk patients with melanoma and the status of metastatic disease. In addition, the emerging availability of specific measures of host response to melanoma—both serological (see Livingston, Chapter 6) and cellular (see Storkus et al., Chapter 7)—offers new modalities that may prove to be critical determinants of disease outcome in the future.

The prognosis of clinically localized melanoma can be stablished to reasonable precision on the basis of the depth of the primary tumor lesion and the clinical or pathological status of regional lymph nodes, as summarized in the TNM classification system and codified in the staging system of the American Joint Commission on Cancer (AJCC). Primary cutaneous melanoma of intermediate Breslow depths of invasion [e.g., between 1.5 and 4.0 mm (T_3, AJCC stage IIA)] have an overall risk of relapse that approaches 30% at 3 years and 40–50% at 5 years (Fig. 1). This group has an *intermediate*

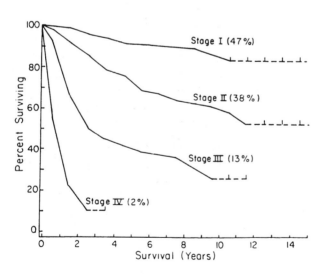

FIGURE 1 Survival according to AJCC stage (% of patients presenting at each stage).

risk of relapse and death in comparison to patients with the thinnest T_1 lesions < 0.76 mm or T_2 tumors < 1.50 mm. Melanoma localized to the skin with a Breslow depth > 4 mm (T_4, AJCC stage IIB) has a relapse rate of >50% at 5 years and approaches the risk profile of patients with regional lymph node involvement. The presence of regional lymph node involvement or the presence of "in-transit" lymphatic metastases between the primary site and regional draining lymph nodes defines groups of patients with relapse rates over 70% at 5 years. These groups have therefore been characterized as groups at *high* relapse risk. The results obtained in preclinical studies of a variety of immunological approaches suggest that their greatest effect is in the setting of low tumor burden, leading to the adjuvant exploration of multiple immunological agents ranging from microbial immunostimulants such as BCG and OK432, and chemical immunomodulators such as levamisole, to the recombinant cytokines and interferons, as well as vaccines (as discussed by Storkus et al., Chapter 7, and Livingston, Chapter 6). Against this argument for the evaluation of immunological approaches in lower- and intermediate-risk groups is the more favorable prognosis for patients with thinner, node-negative, "intermediate-risk" T_3 and T_2 disease, those for whom the risk of relapse and death may be too low to allow the demonstration of significant benefit from new therapies even if the agent were to be active. These considerations have led initial investigators to focus the design of IFNα2 trials on high-risk patients, although several trials are now maturing in the more heterogeneous intermediate-risk categories of melanoma. A further element of complexity in this issue relates to the performance of sentinel lymph node mapping and selective lymphadenectomy. During the past 5 years, it has been recognized that staging can be refined according to sentinel node mapping and other criteria (7,8). Future trials of adjuvant therapy will need to anticipate the improved prognostic acumen of current surgical evaluation with sentinel

node mapping. Although the design of prospective randomized trials in the past decade has utilized criteria of clinical
staging on the one hand and elective regional lymph node
dissection on the other, both may fail to detect regional
lymph node involvement. No adjuvant trial reported to date
has consistently utilized the sentinel node mapping techniques as the basis for selection of patients for trial. The multicenter selective lymphadenectomy trial (D. Morton, PI) will
be completed in the next year and may guide further investigations as it is analyzed.

III. INTERFERONS (IFNs)

Interferon has been investigated more thoroughly than any
other medical agent for the adjuvant therapy of melanoma.
The genes encoding IFNs of multiple species have been
cloned, expressed, and applied for industrial production since
1981. The IFN studies discussed in this chapter have largely
utilized IFN produced by recombinant DNA technology in the
U.S. and European economic communities over the past 15
years. Early studies of IFNs derived from buffy coat leukocytes (Hu IFNα Le), lymphoblasts (Hu IFNα Ly) and fibroblasts (Hu IFNβ) were seminal contributions to the field.
However, the limited quantity, homogeneity, and biological
consistency of IFN from these sources posed insurmountable
problems for the development of appropriate large-scale trials in multicenter cooperative groups. The American Cancer
Society Task Force on Interferon was instrumental in bring-
ing a series of studies in melanoma, renal cell carcinoma,
lymphoma, and breast cancer to completion in the late 1970s,
and served to stimulate broader industrial pursuit of recombinant IFN at higher dosages for longer periods, first at single institutions and then in multicenter cooperative groups
across the world.

The rationale for the systemic investigation of recombinant rIFNa2 for therapy of patients with melanoma was drawn from the preclinical observations of potent antiproliferative, immunomodulatory, and cell surface antigen-regulating activities and the therapeutic implications of these activities in melanoma (Table 1). It has been recognized more recently that the IFNs have potent antivascular effects, and effects upon antigenic-presenting dendritic cells that may also relate to their antitumor effects (9,10).

The results of early phase I dose-seeking trials of IFNa2 (IFNa2a, Hoffman-La Roche; IFNa2b, Schering-Plough Oncology Biotechnology; and IFNa2c, Boehringer-Ingelheim) demonstrated objective antitumor remissions in 15–20% of patients with metastatic unresectable melanoma. Up to one-third of these responses have been reported to be durable in

TABLE 1

Pleiotropic Activity of the Interferons: Direct, Indirect, and Composite Effects Relevant to Melanoma Therapy

Direct	Immunomodulatory	Antiangiogenic/ vascular
Antiproliferative	Effector cell activation/	Growth factor/
Differentiative	regulation:	receptor
Antiviral	Macrophage/dendritic	modulation
2'5' Oligo A	cell	?(bFGF)/FGFR$_1$
synthetase	Large granular	TGFα/EGFR
Protein kinase	lymphocyte	Integrin modulation
Endonuclease	T cell	?αvβ3
RNase L	B cell	
	Antigen regulation	
	MHC class I	
	MHC class II cell	
	surface antigens	
	Costimulatory molecule	
	CD80, CD86	
	Tumor-restricted cell surface	
	antigens	

several independent series at different centers. Antitumor responses with IFNa2 during the phase I trials were observed more frequently the smaller the burden of disease. This obverse relationship between response and the bulk of disease (reviewed in Ref. 11) suggests the greatest benefit of IFN therapy in patients without clinically apparent disease but with high relapse risk. Patients with deep T_4 stage IIB or node-positive stage III melanoma are nonetheless at 50–80% risk of relapse after surgery and might afford an optimal group for evaluation of the potential antiproliferative, immunological, vascular, and other mechanisms of this agent. As the first positive data have become available from the trials of IFNa2 in the highest-risk cohorts of patients, several groups have undertaken the evaluation of potential benefit of this drug in earlier-stage, lower-risk populations. A further extrapolation of this approach would be to the prevention of melanoma. Trials evaluating the potential impact of IFN on precursors of melanoma, including some of the molecular and immunological features described as potential progression markers of the atypical/dysplastic nevus, have recently been initiated. The application of IFNs for melanoma prevention lies beyond the scope of this chapter; however, the findings of adjuvant trials in high-risk disease will inform both the applications in intermediate-risk disease and prevention.

IV. ADJUVANT CLINICAL EXPERIENCE WITH IFN

The adjuvant trials conducted with IFNa2 discussed here are divided according to the categories of risk of tumor relapse in the treated populations as described above, and according to the species and dosage of therapy tested. The trials of adjuvant IFN therapy in resected melanoma that have been published or reported to date are summarized in Table 2.

TABLE 2

Adjuvant IFNα-2 and γ in High-Risk T_3-T_4/Clinically Node (+) Resected Melanoma (AJCC Stage IIB/III)

Cooperative group/PI	Eligible subjects	N	Investigational treatment	Significant study impact on disease-free (DS) or overall (OS) survival
ECOG 1684/ Kirkwood	T_4, N_1	287	IFNα-2b 20 MU/m²/day IV 5 days/wk × 1 mo + 10 MU/m² SC TIW for 11 mo	DFS(+) OS(+) @ 7 yr
NCCT 83-7052/ Creagan	T_{3-4}, N_1	262	IFNα-2a 20 MU/m²/day IM TIW × 3 mo	DFS(−) OS(−) @ 7 yr
SWOG 8642/ Meyskins	T_{3-4}, N_1	134	IFN g 0.2 mg/day SC QD × 1 yr	DFS(−) OS(−)
EORTC 18871/ Kleeberg	T_{3-4}, N_1	800	IFNα-2a 1 MU/day SC QD × 1 yr vs. IFNγ 0.2 mg/day SC QD × 1 yr	Closed 1996
WHO #16/ Cascinelli	N_{1-2}	444	IFNα-2a 3 MU/day SC TIW × 3 yr	DFS(±)@22 mo DFS(−)OS(−)@39 mo
ECOG 1690/ Kirkwood	T_4, N_1	644	IFNα-2b 20 MU/m²/day IV 5 days/wk × 1 mo + 10 MU/m² SC TIW × 11 mo vs. 3 MU/day SC TIW × 2 yr	Closed 1995
EORTC 18952/ Eggermont	N_1	1000	IFNα-2b 10 MU SC QD 5 days/wk × 1 mo +10 MU SC TIW × 1 yr vs. 10 MU SC/day × 1 mo + 5 MU SC TIW × 2 yr vs. observation	Ongoing
ECOG 1694/ Kirkwood	T_4, N_1	851	IFNα-2b 20 MU/m²/day IV 5 days/wk × 1 mo + 10 MU/m² SC TIW × 11 mo vs. GMK vaccine	Ongoing

V. EASTERN COOPERATIVE ONCOLOGY GROUP HIGH-DOSE IFNα2b HIGH-RISK MELANOMA TRIAL (E1684)

E1684 accrued 287 patients, and detailed analyses of this trial were based on the 280 noncancelled patients for whom complete toxicity and outcome data are available. Patients who entered this trial were randomized to receive standard treatment (observation) or IFNα2b (Intron A, Schering-Plough) at maximum tolerable dosages for 1 year. We anticipated a median relapse-free survival of approximately 1 year, and selected the duration of treatment on this basis, as well as the realization that the tolerance of treatment was not likely to exceed 1 year at high dosage, based on prior experience in metastatic disease. Therapy was designed to be given by the intravenous (IV) route for the first months, followed by the subcutaneous (SC) route for the balance of the interval, for reasons summarized in Table 3.

Initial therapy with high-dose IFNα2b administered by the IV route was selected for the attainment of peak levels with acceptable toxicity and the absence of antibody formation associated with the use of the IV route during our prior

TABLE 3
Rationale for Induction (IV) and Maintenance (SC) Phases
of IFNα2b Therapy

IV induction	SC maintenance
Peak levels: >1000 U/ml attainable only IV	Sustained blood levels best achieved SC
Kinetics: rapid clearance IV, no accumulation	Kinetics allow QOD administration
Toxicity acute but not cumulative	Regimen compatible with home administration/resumption
Antibody response to IV IFNα2b negligible (?tolerance)	of routine activities

phase I studies (12,13). The practical limitations of daily IV therapy administration in the outpatient office led to the choice of alternate-daily (TIW) SC therapy for the balance of 1 year (i.e., 48 weeks) of this regimen.

High-risk patients considered eligible for this trial were defined as those with either $T_4 N_0$ AJCC stage IIB or any T N_1 stage III resected melanoma. These groups were selected as the most consistently definable high-risk candidates as the trial was designed in 1983–84. To enforce balance between the treatment arms, stratification of patients was performed at randomization according to clinical and pathological criteria of nodal involvement with elective lymphadenectomy in all patients who entered this trial. Entry criteria were the presence of primary lesions of T_4 depth, without regional lymph node involvement (group I), or primary lesions of any depth with nonpalpable but pathologically proven regional lymph node involvement (group II), or clinical and pathological involvement at initial presentation (group III). or at subsequent relapse (group IV). Patients with clinically apparent disease extending beyond the capsule of the node at operation, including matting or soft tissue extension, were excluded from this trial. This is to be contrasted to the population studied in WHO Trial #16, discussed below, where evidence of extracapsular extension of disease was noted in nearly half of the subjects. Beyond the complete balance assured by stratified randomization in these four pathologically established disease stage groups, there was excellent balance between the treatment and observation groups for all other factors recognized as relevant prognostic variables at the time of study design. The number of lymph nodes involved by tumor was not enumerated in E1684, and is not reliably possible to evaluate retrospectively, but the size of the trial and the process of randomization in the previously noted strata are reasonable assurance of balance in terms of tumor-involved node numbers. The sequel trial E1690 was stratified according to the number of lymph nodes pathologically involved with tumor.

The outcome of E1684 was first unblinded in 1993 at a median follow-up of 5 years, and first published in 1996 at a mature median follow-up duration of 7 years (5). A significant improvement in both median relapse-free (1.72 vs. 0.98 years) and overall survival (3.82 vs. 2.78 years) was noted in an analysis by intention-to-treat, including all 280 subjects with full follow-up. The E1684 IFNα2b regimen has shown consistent and highly significant results in terms of relapse-free survival over time, with p = 0.001–0.004 in group sequential analyses that were conducted between 1990 and 1993, and an improvement of the continuous relapse-free survival of treated patients that is 42% above that of the observation group (37% vs. 26% at 5 years). Analysis of the trial according to the stratification groups reveal a highly consistent effect in all three node-positive strata (groups II–IV). A treatment interaction in the smallest group of 31 node-negative patients (I) was associated with an imbalance in the distribution of patients with ulcerated primary tumors, a key prognostic factor for patients without nodal involvement. This imbalance and the small size of this stratification group confound further analysis of outcome in this stratum, for which no treatment benefit was observed (p = NS). Primary tumor ulceration was balanced in its distribution in treatment and observation groups for the trial overall and would have been expected to have a prognostic importance secondary to the presence of nodal disease in all other groups. All of the larger node-positive subgroups consistently derived a benefit from IFN treatment, and treatment benefit was most significant for the group with lymph node involvement occurring synchronously at presentation with cutaneous primary melanoma (group III). An analysis of the aggregate of the three node-positive populations, requested by the Oncologic Drug Advisory Committee to the U.S. Food and Drug Administration, demonstrated a highly significant impact of this treatment in terms of both relapse-free survival (p < 0.001) and overall survival (p = 0.006). These data, as analyzed at 7 years, are shown in Figure 2. Toxicity of this regi-

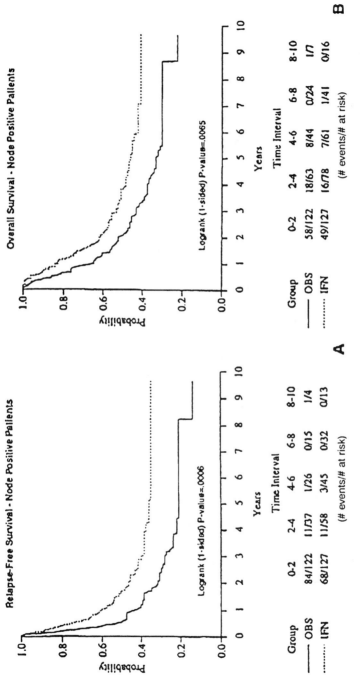

FIGURE 2 (A) Relapse-free and (B) overall survival of node-positive patients on high-dose IFNα2b therapy, at 6.9 years' median follow-up.

men was notable but tolerable, with dose modifications as specified in the original protocol, in the majority (74%) of patients who did not relapse to 1 year. The several major categories of toxicity encountered included constitutional (flu-like), hematological (cytopenic), and hepatic enzyme elevations (Table 4).

The constitutional toxicity associated with IFNα2b encompassed the range of symptoms associated with viral flu-like syndromes. These symptoms were observed to a severe degree at some time in half of subjects treated in E1684. Hematological toxicity of severe (grade 3) or worse degree was observed in almost 25% of patients during treatment. Hepatotoxicity, manifest in enzyme elevations of severe or worse degree (>10× upper limit) was encountered in less than 15% of subjects. Toxicity required delay of treatment or reduction of treatment dosage in more than one-third of patients during the initial month of IV therapy, with subsequent dose delay and/or reduction in similar fraction of patients during the following 11 months of maintenance therapy. Most dose modifications and discontinuations of therapy due to toxicity occurred early during treatment in

TABLE 4

Toxic Events by Type and Degree
(% of 143)

Type	Grade				
	1	2	3	4	5
Constitutional[a]	12.9	37.0	44.8	3.5	0.0
Myelosuppression	25.9	39.9	23.8	0.0	0.0
Hepatotoxicity	21.0	27.3	14.0	0.0	1.4
Neurological	21.7	32.9	23.1	4.9	0.0
Worst grade/pt	1.4	21.0	67.1	9.1	1.4

[a]Worst grade of any constitutional toxicity including fever, chill, and flu-like symptoms: fatigue, malaise, diaphoresis.

this protocol (before the fourth month). In overview, toxicity was the basis for discontinuation of treatment in only one-quarter of patients, and it is notable that the participants in E1684 had no knowledge of the benefit associated with this therapy at the time of their treatment. The two early deaths associated with therapy at 1–3 months in this study both represented hepatotoxicity in patients with incompletely defined prior liver disorders (one viral and one alcoholic), and neither of these patients had been followed according to the stipulated schedule for routine evaluation of liver functions on treatment. Since the importance of close serial evaluation of laboratory parameters (weekly during the first month, monthly × 3, then quarterly for the balance of the year) was initially emphasized to the cooperative group, no further instances of life-threatening liver toxicity have been encountered in either E1684 ($n = 287$) or the subsequent intergroup corroborative trial E1690 ($n = 644$).

In July 1995, the U.S. Food and Drug Administration Oncologic Drug Advisory Committee reviewed the efficacy and safety of IFNα2b as given in E1684 for high-risk melanoma. In December 1995, this therapy was approved for the prevention of relapse and death due to high-risk melanoma, in both $T_4 N_0$ stage IIB patients and node-positive stage III patients, regardless of primary tumor depth. A confirmatory trial (E1690) had already completed accrual in the U.S. Intergroup comparing the high-dose E1684 regimen to a low-dose SC regimen (3 MU SC TIW) given for 2 years, in comparison to observation alone. For this subsequent trial, the prior universal requirement of lymphadenectomy staging of patients for E1684 was dropped, since T_4 (stage IIB) patients were judged to be at sufficient risk to warrant study, regardless of the presence or absence of nodal involvement. This removal of the requirement of surgical staging has led to an enlargement of the fraction of 11% of accrual with node-negative stage IIB disease in E1684, to more than 25% with $T_4 cN_0$ ("IIB") risk profile. The results of the E1690 trial are anticipated to be unblinded in 1998 and will allow a larger series of patients in whom to examine the effects of the high-dose regimen, one with a substantially larger ocmponent with T_4 cN_0 risk.

VI. NORTH CENTRAL CANCER TREATMENT GROUP (NCCTG) 83-7052: ABBREVIATED-COURSE, HIGH-DOSE IFNα2

At the same time tht the IV and SC regimens of maximally tolerable dosage IFNα2b were being developed in our unit in the early 1980s, the Mayo Clinic had gained experience with high- and intermediate-dose IFNα2a administered by the intramuscular (IM) route, demonstrating that durable complete responses were also induced in metastatic melanoma using this regimen. The NCCTG conducted a randomized trial of high doses of IFNα2a (Roche) given IM for 3 months versus observation. This trial, NCCTG 83-7052, enrolled patients with primary cutaneous melanoma < 1.69 mm deep (T_3*, or AJCC stage IIA*/B) or with regional lymph node involvement, concurrent or metachronous. The dose of IFNα2a used was 20 MU/M^2 IM TIW given for 12 weeks. The overall analysis of the outcome of this trial has recently been reported, revealing an absence of benefit upon either relapse-free or overall survival. Analysis of the node-positive (AJCC stage III) patient subset entered into this trial is notable for a trend toward benefit in this subset as analyzed by Cox multivariate techniques. Unfortunately, the limited numbers of node-positive (stage III) patients entered on this trial (n = 162) did not achieve nominal statistical significance for either an impact upon overall or relapse-free survival. The group of patients with more favorable node-negative, intermediate-high-risk IIA*/B melanoma (n = 100) appeared to derive no benefit from this therapy, but the size of this sample is too small to test the question of therapeutic benefit for lower-risk melanoma. This apparent lack of benefit among the most favorable patient subset in this trial is not readily explained, but may reflect an imbalance in the distribution of risk factors such as ulceration. The apparent lack of benefit for stage II patients in both ECOG 1684 and NCCT 83-7052 highlights the statistical requirements for greater numbers when testing for a treatment impact in populations with relatively more favorable disease. The theoretical possibilities for improvement upon the results by prolongation of this IM regimen to achieve a greater benefit have not been explored, but toxicities encountered in the majority of patients treated to 3 months limit this option, as they limit the potential to improve upon the results of E1684 by prolongation of the therapy. The differing dosage, route, initial schedule, duration, and species of agent utilized must be considered, along with the issues of trial design already noted, in comparing the results of the two studies.

VII.   LOW-DOSE IFNα2a IN HIGH-RISK MELANOMA

The WHO Melanoma Programme Trial #16 was developed to test less toxic dosages of IFN that would potentially be tolerable for prolonged periods of time. Treatment for longer than 3 years was initially deliberated, but the final decision was made to test the effect of treatment for 3 years with a low-dose regimen (3 MU SC TIW) of IFNα2a, a dose identical to the low-dose arm of ECOG 1690 (which used IFNa2b for 2 years) versus observation. The patient population studied in WHO Trial #16 (n = 444) was entirely comprised of patients with node-positive disease. Preliminary results of this trial were reported in an early subset analysis at 22 months of median follow-up, suggesting benefit among women > 50 years of age, and men older than 50 years (14). This has not been borne out on reanalysis of the results at 39 months' median follow-up, as presented to the American Society of Clinical Oncology (ASCO) in 1995 and, more recently, as presented to the 4th World Health Congress on Melanoma (Sydney, June 1997) (15). There is presently neither evidence of a meaningful impact upon relapse-free survival, nor any suggestion of survival benefit, with low-dose IFN. A major difference between WHO Trial #16 and the foregoing U.S. cooperative group trials relates to the extent of regional lymph node involvement considered eligible for treatment, as already discussed. Extracapsular extension was permitted in WHO Trial #16, and reported to be present in half of the subjects, whereas E1684 and ECOG 1690, as well as the NCCTG trials already discussed, excluded patients with gross extracapsular extension. Thus, the analysis of WHO Trial #16 and the differences that exist between it and the positive results of the E1684 study must take into account the substantial differences in the trial entry eligibility, as well as the dose, route, schedule, and duration of treatment employed.

VIII.   IFNγ IN INTERMEDIATE- AND HIGH-RISK MELANOMA

Recombinant IFNγ differs significantly from each of the rIFNα2 species, as native IFNγ does from IFNα and IFNβ in its chromosomal gene location, its amino acid content, and interaction with a distinct cell surface receptor—with consequent signal transduction. These elements of distinction between IFNγ and IFNα have recently been elaborated (11). It is notable that IFNγhas exhibited greater immunomodulatory activity as compared with IFNα, where standardized in terms of antiviral activity. On this basis, it was presumed to be a more likely effective immumodulator in vivo, and was therefore subjected to a series of early trials in whch immunomodulatory function upon macrophage/monocyte, NK cell, and T cell was determined (16–18). IFNγ has been licensed for therapy of chronic granulomatous disease, but in multiple trials has shown little antitumor activity as a systemic agent for metastatic disease even in the most extensive dose-response trials, as recently reported by the ECOG (19). Despite this, it had been rapidly brought to trial in the adjuvant setting by the Southwest Oncology Group (SWOG S8642) initiated in 1986 and by the European organization for Research and Treatment of Cancer a year later (EORTC 18871). Patients with intermediate or deep primary melanomas and/or regional lymph node metastases were randomized within 28 days after resection to receive alternate-day therapy with IFNγ SC at a dose of 0.2 mg/day or observation. The study was closed in 1989 after accrual of 284 patients, at which time it was noted that treated patients had both an earlier distribution and an increased frequency of relapse. An early report was issued to this effect, leading to the termination of plans for broader evaluation of this dose schedule of IFNγ therapy in the NCI-Canada (20). However, the adverse trend for the recipients of IFNγ as compared to observation were not then statistically significant, nor at final report has a significant effect been apparent (21). The EORTC trial 18871 compared IFNγ at the same dose schedule tested by SWOG versus IFNα2b at very low doses of 1 MU TIW for 1 year or observation. The results of this trial reveal neither a benefit nor an adverse impact of either intervention as tested in this study (U. Kleeberg, personal communication).

IX. MULTICENTER STUDIES OF IFN IN INTERMEDIATE-RISK, NODE-NEGATIVE MELANOMA

The median depth of incident melanoma has fallen in association with public education campaigns in a number of developed countries (22), and the fraction of deep primary melanoma cases is dwarfed by the intermediate-risk group that is clinically node-negative with Breslow depth 1.5–4.0 mm (T_3, N_0, M_0, stage IIA AJCC). Relapse remains a significant problem for 20–40% of this group of patients, and the relapse risk corresponds directly with Breslow depth and the presence of ulceration, as well as other simple demographic (age, gender, site) and histopathological (mitotic rate and lymphoid infiltrate) factors as variables recently formulated in an index of prognosis (6). The impact of new techniques of lymphatic mapping and sentinel lymph node staging will be felt to the greatest extent in this group of patients, as discussed by Reintgen and Brobeil (Chapter 4) (8). The standard of care for intermediate-risk melanoma has been observation, without good evidence in multiple randomized, controlled trials to argue for elective node dissection or systemic adjuvant therapy. However, the intraoperative sentinel lymph node dye marking technique of Morton et al. (23), in conjunction with the older technique of isotopic lymphoscintigraphy, adds a level of precision to lymph node assessment that has displaced conventional elective lymph node staging. The results of sentinel lymph node mapping and selective lymph node dissection appear to have resolved the heterogeneity of lymph node relapse risk in stage IIA (T_3-N_0) and IIB (T_4-N_0) populations, and may now pose new questions for the subgroups with IIA sentinel node-negative (more favorable), and IIA sentinel node-positive, or sentinel-defined stage III (N_1) disease. For the group in the latter category who have only one node shown to be positive, one may consider the potential option to intervene more effectively and with less morbidity to perform surgical lymph node staging, with systemic medical adjuvant therapy. For sentinel node-negative patients, the risk may be diminished such that a more favorable subgrouping is warranted. The intermediate-risk group may benefit either from ongoing trials of IFNa2 or from a series of ongoing and planned vaccine trials, in part detailed in the chapters of Livingston et al. (see Chapter 6), and Storkus et al. (see Chapter 7).

Table 5 summarizes a series of trials directed at the intermediate-risk category of stage IIA/T_3 melanoma. Groups of investigators in France, Austria, and Scotland have under-

TABLE 5

Trials of IFNα2b and Vaccines in Intermediate Risk T_3-T_4/Clinically Node (–) Resected Melanoma (AJCC Stage IIA-B)

Study	Eligibility	No.	Treatment agent/ dosage/duration	Relapse/ survival impact
SWOG 9035	T_3-T_4, N_0	600		
Austrian (Pehamberger)	T_3-T_4, N_0 IIA-B	~311	IFNα2b, 3 MU SC TIW, 18 mo	TE
French (Grob et al. 1996)	T_3-T_4, N_0 IIA-B	493	IFNα2b, 3 MU SC TIW, 18 mo	RFS (+), OS (–) @ 3 yr
Scottish (Mackie)	T_3-T_4, N_0 IIA-B	~100	IFNα2b, 3 MU SC TIW, 18 mo	TE
ECOG 1697	T_3-T_4, N_0 IIA	1000	IFNα2b, 20 MU/m²/day IV 5 × wk × 4	TE

taken randomized controlled adjuvant trials of low-dose IFNα2b in 300–500 patients with stage IIA T_3,N_0,M_0 melanoma patients each, administered generally at dosages of 3 MU SC TIW for 18 months. The French Multicenter trial, led by J. J. Grob, was initially reported at the American Society of Clinical Oncology, at a median follow-up of 3 years (24). At this early point of assessment, a nominally significant impact was observed upon overall survival, but not relapse-free survival; more recently, at a median follow-up of approximately 5 years, the impact upon overall survival has been reported on longer to be statistically significant (25). As observed in the previously described WHO Trial #16 in stage III melanoma, the pattern of impact of this low-dose regimen is notable for a gradual divergence of relapse event rates between the treated and control populations, with a collapse of the lemon-shaped envelope of divergence after discontinuation of therapy. The benefit, enduring for approximately the interval of therapy, suggests a cytostatic or labile impact upon the disease, and the hazard plot for the initial analysis of the French multicenter trial, like that of WHO Trial #16, reveals a suppression of relapses appearing gradually during therapy, but a loss of this benefit as treatment is withdrawn at 18–36 months (15,24).

The impact of the low-dose IFN regimens studied thus far upon relapse-free survival is encouraging, but the lack of a durable benefit with any published low-dose regimens to date leads to the consideration of vaccine regimens as alternatives for patients at lesser relapse risk. As we have the details of final analyses of the French, Austrian, and Scottish studies conducted since 1990, we will be able to compare the therapeutic impact of these regimens versus vaccines tested to date. These low-dose trials of IFNα2b and IFNα2a have yet to be fully reported in the literature. Therefore, judgment must be withheld at this point. Given the numbers of patients accrued among the several trials, and the similarities of dosage, route, schedule, and patient cohort enrolled, it is obvious that meta-analyses of these treatments may be undertaken.

Given these observations, two alternative strategies suggest themselves: the use of the low-dose IFNα2 therapy for an indefinite period, or the evaluation and development of derivative therapies with higher-dosage IFNα2 modelled upon E1684, but for shorter periods.

It is uncertain what the relative importance of the IV component (20 MU/m^2/day 5 days/wk $\times$ 1 month), as opposed to the S.C. component (10 MU/m^2/day TIW IFN $\times$ 48 weeks) in the efficacy of the E1684 regimen may have been. The toxicity of the entire regimen is beyond what would be reasonable to consider for patients with stage IIA disease. One hypothesis regarding the benefit of E1684 is that this may have derived largely from the effects of the peak doses delivered IV in the initial month. With this rationale in mind, the ECOG has proposed to test the adjuvant therapeutic benefit of just the IV component of E1684 in the stage IIA intermediate-risk category of patients with melanoma (E1697, S. Agarwala and J. Kirkwood, Co-PIs). If, as suggested by the hazard-function analysis, the IV component of E1684 has a durable (cytotoxic or immunomodulatory) effect, the activity of the abbreviated regimen may rival that of the full 1-year program. Accrual to this regimen will continue through the year 2000, and the anticipated analysis of relapse-free survival will be anticipated in the 2–3 years following that.

X. EVALUATION OF INTERMEDIATE ENDPOINTS OF ADJUVANT IFN THERAPIES FOR HIGH-RISK AND INTERMEDIATE-RISK MELANOMA: IMMUNOLOGICAL, QUALITY-OF-LIFE, AND COST ISSUES

The analysis of potential immunological and antiproliferative mechanisms of IFN has been pursued in a parallel prospective laboratory study, E2690, nested within the recent U.S. Intergroup Trial E1690. This laboratory corollary study accrued 139 subjects for serial blood sampling and secured samples of autologous tumor cells from a smaller subset of patients. A variety of phenotypic and functional assays have been performed to evaluate a number of the postulated mechanisms listed in Table 1. The therapeutic trial will be unblinded in 1998 and will then allow the correlation of baseline values and changes over time in relation to high versus low doses of IFN and observation. It is hoped thatn an examination of these mechanisms in relation to subsequent disease course will reveal immunological and/or antitumor functions that correspond with therapeutic response to IFN in terms of relapse-free and overall survival and baseline functions associated with relapse-free survival. At present, comparison of the impact of the high-dose E1684 regimen in high-risk disease and the low-dose regimen in intermediate-risk disease demonstrates a relatively larger reduction in the hazard of death for the high-dose regimen at 5 years (25% vs. 17%) and a difference in the long-term prospect of durable disease-free survival which offers the potential for cure with this therapy.

A curative benefit is achieved with the E1684 regimen in only a subset of patients and, until the results of E2690 (or other studies now in progress) allow us to define the patients destined to benefit from therapy, treatment to benefit the responsive subset must be given to the larger high-risk population. The impact of this regimen on quality of life, therefore, becomes an issue, which has been addressed retrospectively using the E1684 dataset and the "Q-TWiST" methodology of Goldhirsch (26). This analysis compartmentalizes time with toxicity or relapse, apart from disease-free off-treatment time, to quantitate the useful time gained for high-risk patients through therapy. Q-TWiST analysis (27) has demonstrated a benefit that accrues over time and shows a benefit for the majority of patients, even after subtraction of the time during which toxicity of treatment was experienced. Because toxicity is perceived differently by different patients, the analysis must include a weighted factor according to the patient's perception of treatment toxicity. Even for those patients with the most severely compromised quality of life on treatment, a net benefit was demonstrated. The net gain function in quality-adjusted survival for the entire cohort of E1684 analyzed by intent to treat becomes positive, even for those patients with the greatest perceived toxicity, after 6 years. Q-TWiST analysis of the quality-adjusted benefit for patients without significant toxicity is positive from the outset. The quality-adjusted survival time accrued for patients treated with IFN in E1684 analyzed by the Q-TWiST technique is statistically significant for the high-risk, node-positive group of patients treated in E1684.

The issue of cost-efficacy of the therapy tested in E1684 has been reported in two independent analyses: one from

Bologna, Italy, published in the European literature (28), and the other by Hillner et al. in collaboration with the original investigators (29,30). Both analyses have shown remarkably similar conclusions. The Hillner analysis of the E1684 trial compiled the costs of care, including relapse, to calculate costs for both near (7-year) and long-term (35-year) horizons. Both cost-efficacy analyses demonstrate long-term costs per year of life gained or per quality-adjusted year of life gained of $16–18,000. These are well within the range of accepted adjuvant therapies for other solid tumors such as node-positive breast carcinoma and colorectal adenocarcinoma (30,31).

XI. SYNTHESIS OF THE EXPERIENCE WITH IFNα2 ADJUVANT THERAPY: PROSPECTS FOR THE FUTURE

The overall analysis of the results of trials performed with high-dose and low-dose IFNα2 in high-risk melanoma leads to several general conclusions: In high-risk melanoma groups (with either T_4 primary lesions or proven regional lymph node metastasis), the data are currently inconclusive, but support only high-dose therapy administered for 1 year on the basis of the mature E1684 trial. The benefit of this therapy administered beginning within 2 months of surgery is rapidly manifest in terms of reduced relapse rate and death. This benefit is sustained for a median follow-up of more than 7 years, with stable and durable benefit enduring to a point where it is likely that a significant fraction of the treated patients were cured. The toxicity of this regimen is significant but manageable. While the positive results have derived from a single study, this dataset, audited by the ECOG, by the industry, and by the FDA prior to FDA approval, is compelling. The mature significant positive results are unequivocal for the node-positive populations studied, all three groups of whom show highly significant survival and relapse-free benefit. Corroboration of this trial is anticipated from E1690, which will reach maturity and final analysis in 1998. The overall positive results of E1684 and the positive trend reported for the high-risk, node-positive subset of NCCTG 83-7052 argue that the benefit of IFNα2 adjuvant therapy is readily demonstrated among the highest-risk (i.e., node-positive) populations of melanoma, as it has been for chemotherapy in breast and colorectal carcinoma. Melanoma with gross extracapsular extension or matted regional lymph node involvement was not studied in the E1684 trial, but in the low-dose WHO Trial #16 appears not to derive even the early transient benefit noted for relapse-free survival with that regimen. Given the increased regional relapse risk of this category of disease, it would seem logical to investigate combined-modality therapy, including measures directed at the regional tumor burden, such as radiotherapy, in conjunction with systemic measures such as IFNα2b at high dosage. A trial of this design is under development in the U.S. Cooperative Groups at this time (D. Wazer, PI, ECOG Trial 3697).

XII. ALTERNATE REGIMENS OF INTERMEDIATE-DOSAGE IFNα2b

The toxicity of the high-dose E1684 trial, during both the induction period of the first month of IV therapy and the subsequent 11 months of SC maintenance, has led to the pursuit of alternate routes and dose schedules for adjuvant IFN therapy of high-risk postoperative patients with melanoma. A recently commenced EORTC trial—EORTC 18952—tests two intermediate-dose regimens of SC IFNα2b, omitting the initial IV induction phase and adopting an initial month of daily SC therapy at 10 MU/day, followed by 11 months of treatment at 10 MU TIW, or 23 months of treatment at 5 MU TIW, such that cumulative dosages delivered over 1 or 2 years are ultimately equivalent. This trial, directed at high-risk patients, will accrue 400 patients to each of the treatment arms with 200 assigned to observation. The active treatment regimen utilized in E1684 was not included in this trial, so it will be difficult to compare the relative activity of the two intermediate arms against that of E1684. The U.S. Cooperative Groups have recently undertaken a study of the new ganglioside GM2 vaccine (detailed in Livingston, Chapter 6), in comparison to IFNα2b as given in E1684. This trial, E1694/S9512 (J. Kirkwood, PI), will accrue 851 patients with AJCC stage IIB or III over the next 2 years, and is anticipated to reach analysis by the year 2001.

For intermediate-risk melanoma patients, the results of the French multicenter study of Grob et al. are encouraging but still in flux, and the early report of a significant impact on survival has given way to a suggestion of transient prolongation of relapse-free interval without a significant survival benefit (32). The results of low-dose IFNα2a therapy in both intermediate- and high-risk melanoma have shown a gradual appearance of treatment impact upon the frequency of relapse, and a loss of treatment effect after discontinuation of therapy. These suggest a cytostatic effect dependent upon the presence of the agent. In these respects it will be important to determine whether the influence upon earlier T_3 node-negative stage IIA melanoma in the Austrian and Scottish trials differs from the impact upon such patients in the French multicenter trial or the node-positive stage III patients in the WHO #16 trial. The E1690/S9190 Intergroup U.S. trial will provide further evidence in regard to high-risk patients. As these recent trials mature, it will be possible to draw more definitive conclusions.

The analysis of the mechanism of antitumor impact of IFNα2b is critical for progress, and the E2690 corollary may allow the more precise application of IFN to those patients most likely tto benefit from this therapy. At present, it is not possible to conclude whether the benefit derived from IFN is related to direct antiproliferative, differentiative, antivascular, or antigen-regulatory effects—or associated with the modulation of specific antitumor immune responses. As these factors are better elucidated, it will be possible to determine which combined-modality efforts with vaccines will be most fruitful.

XIII. COMBINED APPLICATION OF IFN AND VACCINES

The rapid advance of the field of vaccine therapy for melanoma has led to the development of a series of combined-modality trials for patients with metastatic high- and intermediate-risk disease. In metastatic resectable disease, the whole-cell vaccines pioneered by D. Morton and M. Mitchell are being evaluated in combination with IFN at a range of dosages and in a variety of schedules. For the chemically defined ganglioside GM2 vaccine discussed by Livingston (Chapter 6), the ECOG has developed both a phase III trial (E1694) for stage IIB-III disease and a phase II trial for patients with high-risk disease ineligible for E1694 (E2696). The latter trial tests the interaction of IFNα2b at high dosage given concurrently with, or beginning 1 month after, the initiation of vaccine vs. vaccine alone in patients with resectable metastatic disease or stage IIB or III disease who do not fit the eligibility criteria for E1694. The endpoint of these trials is the induction of anti-GM2 antibody response, so that the results—defining potential synergism, antagonism, or a lack of interaction—will rapidly permit the development of GM2 vaccine combinations for combined-modality adjuvant therapy. It remains to develop appropriate surrogate markers for the peptide/protein and other vaccines that may permit their evaluation in conjunction with IFNs and other immunomodulators, as discussed elsewhere in this volume. Clearly, each of these modalities will have their greatest potential return as applied to the high-risk adjuvant disease setting in melanoma.

REFERENCES

1. Quirt IC, Shelley WE, Pater JL, Bodurtha AJ, McCulloch PB, McPherson TA, Paterson AHG, Prentice R, Silver HKB, Willan AR, et al. Improved survival in patients with poor prognosis malignant melanoma treated iwth adjuvant levamisole: a phase III study by the National Cancer Institute of Canada Clinical Trials Group. J Clin Oncol 1991; 9(5): 729–735.
2. Spitler LE. A randomized trial of levamisole versus placebo as adjuvant therapy in malignant melanoma. J Clin Oncol 1991; 9(5):736–740.
3. Loutfi A, Shakr A, Jerry M, et al. Double blind randomized prospective trial of levamisole/placebo in stage I cutaneous melanoma. Clin Invest Med 1987; 10:325–328.
4. Lejeune FJ, Macher E, Kleeberg U, Rumke P, Prade M, Thomas D, Suciu S. An assessment of DTIC versus levamisole or placebo in the treatment of high risk stage I patients after surgical removal of a primary melanoma of the skin. A phase II adjuvant study (EORTC protocol 18761). Eur J Cancer 1988; 24:S81–S90.
5. Kirkwood JM, Strawderman MH, Ernstoff MS, Smith TJ, Borden EC, Blum RH. Interferon alfa-2b adjuvant therapy of high-risk resected cutaneous melanoma: the Eastern Cooperative Oncology Group Trial EST 1684. J Clin Oncol 1996; 14:7–17.
6. Schuchter L, Schultz D, Synnestvedt BS, Trock BJ, Guerry D, Elder DE, Elenitsas R, Clark WH, Halpern AC. A prognostic model for predicting 10-year survival in patients with primary melanoma. Ann Intern Med 1996; 125:369–375.
7. Ross MI, Balch CM, Soong S, McCarthy WH, Tinoco L, Mansfield P, Lee JE, Bedikian A, Eton O, Plager C, et al. Critical analysis of the current American Joint Committee on Cancer staging system for cutaneous melanoma and proposal of a new staging system. J Clin Oncol 1997; 15:1039–1051.
8. Reintgen D, Balch CM, Kirkwood JM, Ross M. Recent advances in the care of the patient with malignant melanoma. Ann Surg 1997; 1:1–14.
9. Hanahan D, Folkman J. Patterns and emerging mechanisms

of the angiogenic switch during tumorigenesis. Cell 1996; 86:353–364.

10. Dvorak E. Experimental design for vaccine preparations against human malignant tumors. Med Hypo 1990; 20:428–452.

11. Kirkwood JM. Biologic therapy with interferon α and β: clinical applications—melanoma. In: DeVita VT Jr, Hellman S, Rosenberg SA, eds. Biologic Therapy of Cancer: Principles and Practice. Philadelphia: JB Lippincott, 1996:388–411.

12. Kirkwood JM, Ernstoff MS, Davis CA, Reiss M, Ferraresi R, Rudnick SA. Comparison of intramuscular and intravenous recombinant alpha-2 interferon in melanoma and other cancers. Ann Intern Med 1985; 103(1):32–36.

13. Kirkwood JM. Melanoma. In: Biologic Therapy of Cancer: Principles and Practice. 1994:388–411.

14. Cascinelli N, Bufalino R, Morabito A, MacKie R. Results of adjuvant interferon study in WHO melanoma programme. Lancet 1997; 343:913–914.

15. Cascinelli N. Evaluation of efficacy of adjuvant rIFNα 2A in melanoma patients with regional node metastases. Proc ASCO 1995; 14:A1296 (abstract).

16. Kirkwood JM, Ernstoff MS, Trautman T, Hebert G, Nishida Y, Davis CA, Balzer J, Reich S, Schindler J, Rudnick SA. In vivo biological response to recmobinant interferon gamma during a phase I dose-response trial in patients with metastatic melanoma. J Clin Oncol 1990; 8(6):1070–1082.

17. Urba WJ, Kopp WC, Clark JW, Smith JW, Steis RG, Huber C, Cogin D, Longo DL. The in vivo immunomodulatory effects of recombinant interferon gamma plus recombinant tumor necrosis factor-alfa. J Clin Oncol1991; 9:1831–1839.

18. Kirkwood JM, Bryant J, Schiller JH, Strawderman MH, Borden EC, Whiteside TL. Immunomodulatory function of interferon gamma in patients with metastatic melanoma: results of a phase I trial in subjects with metastatic melanoma (EST 4987). J Immunother 1997; 20(2):146–157.

19. Schiller JH, Pugh M, Kirkwood J. Phase II/III trial of interferon-gamma in metastatic melanoma: an innovative trial design. Clin Cancer Res 1996; 2:29–36.

20. Meyskens FL, Jr., Kopecky K, Samson M, Hersh E, MacDon-

ald J, Jaffe H, Crowley J, Coltman C. Recombinant human interferon gamma; adverse effects in high-risk stage I and II cutaneous malignant melanoma. J Natl Cancer Inst 1990; 82(12):1071.

21. Meyskens FL, Kopecky KJ, Taylor CW, Noyes RD, Tuthill RJ, HErsh EM, Feun LG, Doroshow JH, Flaherty LE, Sondak VK. Randomized trial of adjuvant human interferon gamma versus observation in high-risk cutaneous melanoma: a Southwest Oncology Group Study. J Natl Cancer Inst 1995; 87:1070–1713.

22. Mackie RM, Hole DJ. Incidence and thickness of primary tumours and survival of patients with cutaneous malignant melanoma in relation to socioeconomic status. Br Med J 1996; 312:1125–1128.

23. Morton DL, Foshag LJ, Hoon DS, Nizze JA, Wanek LA, Chang C, Davtyan DG, et al. Prolongation of survival in metastatic melanoma after active specific immunotherapy with a new polyvalent melanoma vaccine. Ann Surg 1992; 463–482.

24. Grob JJ, Dreno B, Delaunay M, Chastang C, Guillot B, Cupissol B, Souteyrand P, Sassolsas B, Cesarini JP, Thivolet J, et al. Results of the French multicenter trial on adjuvant therapy with interferon alfa-2a in resected primary melanoma (<1.5mm). Proc ASCO 1996; 15:437.

25. Kirkwood JM. Interferon alpha to be as adjuvant therapy for high-risk melanoma. Melanoma Res 1997; 7:S23 (abstract).

26. Gelber RD, Goldhirsch A, Cole BF. Evaluation of effectiveness: q-twist. Cancer Treat Rev 1993; 19:73–84.

27. Cole BF, Gelber RD, Kirkwood JM, Goldhirsch A, Barylak E, Borden E. A quality-of-life-adjusted survival anaysis of interferon alfa-2b adjuvant treatment for high-risk resected cutaneous melanoma: an Eastern Cooperative Oncology Group Study (E1684). J Clin Oncol1996; 14:2666–2673.

28. Messori A, Becagli P, Trippoli S. Cost-effectiveness of interferon-alpha as maintenance therapy in chronic myelogenous leukemia. Ann Intern Med 1997; 126:664–665.

29. Hillner BE, Kirkwood JM, Atkins MB, Johnson ER, Smith TJ. Economic analysis of adjuvant interferon alfa-2b in high-risk melanoma based on projections from ECOG 1684. J Clin Oncol1997. In press.

30. Hillner BE, Kirkwood JM. Economic analyses of benefit from interferon-alfa2B in high risk melanoma: tradeoffs between completeness, simplicity, and clarity. Eur J Cancer 1997. In press.
31. Smith TJ, Hillner BE, Mitchell RB. Decision analysis in non-small-cell lung cancer: not back to the (drawing) modeling board, back to the bedside. J Clin Oncol 1997; 15:870–872.
32. Grob JJ, Dreno B, Delaunay M, et al. Long term results of an adjuvant therapy with low doses IFN-alpha2A in resected primary melanoma thicker than 1.5 mm without clinically detectable node metastases. Melanoma Res 1997; 7:S33 (abstract).

6

THE CASE FOR MELANOMA VACCINES THAT INDUCE ANTIBODIES

Philip O. Livingston

Memorial Sloan-Kettering Cancer Center
New York, New York

I. RATIONALE FOR ACTIVE SPECIFIC IMMUNOTHERAPY OF MELANOMA WITH VACCINES

A sound basis exists for the development of melanoma vaccines. First, there is the dramatic success of vaccines against infectious diseases: while these vaccines have generally been used for protection from future infections, some have also been shown to be effective when administered after exposure (2,3). Second, cancer vaccines protect against experimental tumors in rodents and, in some cases, mediate regression of established syngeneic cancers (4,5). As well, a variety of whole melanoma-cell or cell-lysate vaccines have induced occasional significant tumor responses in melanoma patients over the last 25 years (18–21; reviewed in 22,41). The frequency of these responses is too high to be attributed to spontaneous remissions that are seen in melanoma patients on rare occasions. Melanoma antigens have been defined on human melanomas using antibodies, helper T cells, and cytotoxic T cells obtained from melanoma patients. Qualitative and quantitative differences between melanoma cells and most normal cells have been demonstrated. The presence of antibodies or cytotoxic T cells against some of these antigens in melanoma patients correlates with a more favorable prognosis (6–8). Partial or complete clinical responses have been reported in a proportion of melanoma patients treated with monoclonal antibodies or tumor-infiltrating lymphocytes that react with these antigens (9–13). Moreover, antibody and T-cell responses against some of these well-defined tumor antigens can be augmented by tumor vaccines (14–17; modified from 1).

II. RATIONALE FOR THE CONSTRUCTION OF CANCER VACCINES THAT INDUCE ANTIBODIES

The role of T lymphocytes in mediating tumor rejection is widely known and accepted. The importance of B lymphocytes and antibodies in this setting is less well recognized. With regard to immunity against bacteria, complement mediated effector mechanisms (opsonification and lysis) are known to correlate with protection. The relevant mechanisms involved in antibody mediated rejection of cancer have not been defined. However, passive immunotherapy by administration of monoclonal antibodies has resulted in resistance to tumor challenge and regression of a variety of experimental solid tumors (see Table 1). The protective effect is consistently greatest when the monoclonal antibodies are administered within 24–48 hours of the tumor challenge, timing which may be comparable to the adjuvant setting in humans.

Regression of detectable cancers has also been accomplished in humans following treatment with monoclonal antibodies against gangliosides, HER2/neu glycoprotein, and

TABLE 1

Basis for Cancer Vaccines that Induce Antibody Responses: Passive Immunotherapy of Solid Tumors in Rodents Giving ≥ 50% Protection

Antibody (antigen)	Route[a] mAb	Challenge	Cancer type	Ref.
TA99 (gp75)	IP	IV	B16F10 melanoma	23
T97, 2-3-1 (B700)	IV	IV	JB/MS melanoma	24
Clone A8 (MMTV)	IP	SC	H2712 mammary cancer	25
R24 (GD3)	IP	SC	Ab hamster melanoma	—[b]
8F11 (αplt. aggr.)	IV	IV	NL-17 (colon 26) murine colon ca.–nude	26
e21+23 (erb B-2)	IP	SC	N87 human gastric ca.–nude	27
4D5 (erb B-2)	IV	SC	4-IST human gastric ca.–scid	28
BR96 (Le[y] variant)	IV	SC	H2707 human lung ca.–nude	29
225 (EGFR)	IP	SC	A431 human ca.–nude	30

[a]Antibody administration started 1–10 days after tumor challenge.
[b]Paul Chapman, M.D. (Memorial Sloan-Kettering Cancer Center, New York, NY), personal communication.

immunoglobulin idiotypes (see Table 2). In addition, passive immunotherapy of colon cancer in the adjuvant setting with monoclonal antibody CO17-A has prolonged disease-free and overall survival (36).

Active immunotherapy by immunization with protein or glycoprotein tumor antigens results in a complex immune response, making it difficult to determine the role of antibodies in the resulting protection. Carbohydrate tumor antigens, however, are known to mediate a predominantly if not exclusively antibody response. Vaccination with carbohydrate tumor antigens has resulted in evidence for protection from tumor challenge and tumor regression in experimental animals and protection from melanoma recurrence in humans (see Table 3).

Drawing on evidence concerning the role of antibodies in protection against various infectious diseases, the presumed role of antibodies in immunotherapy of cancer is the induction of complement mediated opsonification and cytotoxicity against circulating tumor cells and micrometastases. Improved antigen presentation of melanoma protein and glycoprotein antigens to T lymphocytes by B lymphocytes and other professional antigen-presenting cells following anti-

TABLE 2

Basis for Cancer Vaccines that Induce Antibody Responses:
Passive Immunotherapy in Humans

Antibody (antigen)	mAb route	Cancer type	Response (protection)	Ref.
R24 (GD3)	IV	Melanoma	10%	9,10,11
3F8, 14.G2a, 14.G9a (GD2)	IV	Neuroblastoma	10–30%	31,32,55
L55, L72 (GM2, GD2)	IL	Melanoma	50–100%	33,34
Anti-id mAbs	IV	B-cell lymphoma	55%	35
HER2 (erB-2)	IV	Breast cancer	12%	37
CO17–A (GA733)	IV	Colorectal cancer	(15%)	36

TABLE 3

Basis for Cancer Vaccines that Induce Antibody Responses:
Active Immunotherapy

	Target antigen	Vaccine	Cancer type	Response (protection)	Ref.
Mice	T_N	Cy/T_N-KLH + R$_{IBI}$	TA3-HA	50%	38
	TF	Cy/TF-KLH + R$_{IBI}$	TA3-HA	50% (90%)	39
Man	GM2	GM2/BCG	Melanoma	(12%)	14

body induction and antibody-mediated tumor destruction
may also lead to tumor regression. If antibodies of sufficient
titer can be induced against cell surface tumor antigens to
eliminate tumor cells from the blood and lymphatic system,
and to eradicate micrometastases, this would dramatically
change our approach to treating the cancer patient. With repeated showers of metastases no longer possible, aggressive
local therapies of established cancers, including surgery and
intralesional treatments, might result in long-term control
even of metastatic cancers.

III. OBSTACLES TO THE CONSTRUCTION OF CONSISTENTLY IMMUNOGENIC, CLINICALLY EFFECTIVE MELANOMA VACCINES AND SOLUTIONS

The studies performed with tumor vaccines to date have not
readily translated into vaccines of consistent therapeutic
benefit for the melanoma patient for a variety of reasons (see
Table 4). To begin with, there is little clear evidence that primary or metastatic melanoma induces protective immunity
in patients. Consequently, it has been difficult to demonstrate an association between any particular immune response (surrogate marker) against cancer and delayed

TABLE 4

Obstacles to the Construction of Clinically Effective
Melanoma Vaccines

1. Low immunogenicity of tumor antigens and tolerance.
2. Adjacent antigens on tumor cells provide no help.
3. Uncertainty over the relevant effector mechanisms.
4. Lack of clinically relevant surrogate endpoints.
5. Tumor and host heterogeneity.

recurrence or improved survival. This lack of disease-induced immunity is unlike the picture with most infectious disease where such surrogate immune response markers have been the starting point for construction of successful vaccines. What is needed for the development of successful vaccines against melanoma is a method for rapid assessment of immunogenicity of melanoma antigens which can be used to guide the process of vaccine construction and modification (i.e., to characterize and quantify immune responses to specific antigens and, if possible, to correlate these responses to clinical outcome). The development of vaccines against infectious diseases has relied on serological responses against bacterial or viral antigens and, more recently, T-cell responses, following vaccination. These advances were expedited by the precise definition of immunogenic epitopes of these pathogens. Recent progress in defining immunogenic antigens that are shared by many melanomas, and in augmenting their immunogenicity, has revolutionized melanoma vaccine development. While the quest for reliable surrogate markers of T-cell immunity against melanoma following vaccination is currently the focus of many laboratories, reliable surrogate markers for B-cell immunity against melanoma are already in hand.

There are several additional obstacles. Functional and antigenic heterogeneity are inherent features of melanomas, and genetically based heterogeneity of responsiveness is inherent in the human immune response. Also, most of the melanoma antigens identified have been autoantigens, so active immunization involves overcoming a degree of immunological tolerance. This tolerance is undoubtedly reinforced by the presence of the growing tumor and the increasing quantities of shed antigen, similar to the protection seen against induction of experimental autoimmunity by injection of free antigen prior to the normally pathogenic immunization (40). Finally, it seems likely that normal cell surface antigens adjacent to relevant melanoma antigens are important. Melanoma antigens are poor immunogens, because they are autoantigens and because they are surrounded by autoantigens. In the absence of strong bystander immunogens, the conditions necessary for optimal B- and T-lymphocyte responses to melanoma antigens, such as recruitment and activation of professional antigen-presenting cells and/or cytokine production by T-helper cells, may not be present. On the other hand, the antigens of viral or bacterial pathogens are potent immunogens, not just because they are foreign (nonself) antigens, but also because they are surrounded by other foreign antigens. Sequential purification of even these highly foreign antigens has resulted in progressive decrease in their immunogenicity. It appears that the immune system utilizes the foreign milieu of these antigens to provide help for the immune response against potential pathogens, just as it takes advantage of the normal autoantigen milieu of autoantigens to make immunization more difficult.

Based on these considerations, the design of maximally immunogenic tumor vaccines would ideally include:

1. Taking the antigens out of their normal autoantigen environment and putting them in the context of immunogenic foreign antigens for presentation to the immune system.
2. The use of a potent immunological adjuvant to further augment immunogenicity.

3. Overcoming the issues of tumor and host heterogeneity by early intervention at minimal tumor burden and the use of polyvalent vaccines.
4. Limiting reinforcement of tolerance by vaccinating
early in the disease course, preferably in the adjuvant setting.

IV. PREVIOUS EXPERIENCE WITH MELANOMA VACCINES

Many thousands of melanoma patients have been injected
with a variety of melanoma cell preparations in this country
and elsewhere over the past thirty years, but the design and
complexity of these studies has made an assessment of the
value of this approach to melanoma therapy difficult (22,41;
modified from 1). In the majority of these trials, the cell lines
used for vaccine production had not been selected for maxi-
mal expression of known tumor antigens, and it was unclear
whether, in fact, patients responded immunologically to
melanoma antigens following vaccination, in part because
adequate techniques to measure the immune response were
not available and many tumor antigens were still not known.
The major clinical response rates in a number of these trials
approximated 10–20%, but the vaccines used in the successful trials were poorly characterized, by modern standards,
and the difference in composition from that of the vaccines
used in trials with lower or zero response rates was not apparent. These results demonstrate that active specific immunotherapy of melanoma with vaccines can induce tumor
regression occasionally, but they have failed to provide a
solid foundation for the construction of increasingly effective
vaccines.

A variety of immune responses have been described
following several of these trials. Induction of antibodies
against GM2 ganglioside (6,7,15), the high-molecular-

weight melanoma chondroitin sulfate proteoglycan (42,43), and several incompletely defined antigens (20,44,45) have each been shown to correlate with an improved prognosis. Consequently, each of these serological responses may be appropriate surrogate markers for further clinical trials aimed at augmenting immunogenicity, constructing consistently immunogenic vaccines, and eventually determining the impact of immunization on the clinical course. Studies with GM2 ganglioside are furthest advanced in this regard and so will be reviewed here as an example of the pathway that other antigens (whether recognized by B or T lymphocytes) will follow.

V. SELECTION OF GANGLIOSIDES AS TARGETS FOR VACCINE THERAPY IN MELANOMA PATIENTS

Gangliosides are sialic-acid-containing glycosphingolipids that are overexpressed at the cell surface of cancers of neuroectodermal origin, including melanomas (46,47). Gangliosides GM2, GM3, GD2, GD3, and 9-0 acetyl GD3 are expressed on most melanomas. GM2 has proved to be the most immunogenic of these gangliosides in melanoma patients. The importance of gangliosides as targets for immunotherapy of melanoma has been documented by the immunogenicity of GM2 and GD2; by clinical responses seen after treatment with monoclonal antibodies against GM2, GD2, and GD3; and by a clear correlation between the presence of natural or vaccine-induced IgM antibody against GM2 and improved prognosis (1).

Between 1975 and 1985, Livingston et al. immunized more than 100 patients with a series of melanoma cell vaccines admixed with various adjuvants or viruses and analyzed the resulting immune responses (14,22,41). All patients mounted strong serologic responses against melanoma cells as a consequence of the immunizations. While most of these responses were against artifactual allo- or xeno-antigens such as HLA antigens or fetal calf serum, several responses with relative specificity for melanoma cells were induced. The only melanoma antigens recognized by more than one patient were the gangliosides GM2 and GD2. Tai et al. also found GM2 and GD2 to be particularly immunogenic (48). Hence both active and passive immunotherapy trials have identified ganglioside antigens as uniquely effective targets for cancer immunotherapy.

Based on the occasional anti-GM2 ganglioside antibody responses induced by vaccination with melanoma cells, we explored a variety of vaccines containing purified GM2 ganglioside. GM2 alone was not immunogenic, and GM2 adherent to the surface of *Salmonella minnesota* mutant R595, liposomes or liposome-like structures called proteosomes induced antibody responses in about 50% of patients (14). Of the GM2 vaccines initially studied, purified GM2 adherent to *bacillus Calmette-Guérin* (BCG) was the most consistently immunogenic vaccine, inducing antibodies in 85% of patients (49). Production of the GM2 antibody after immunization was associated with an improved prognosis compared to antibody-negative patients or historical controls.

Consequently, a randomized trial was conducted in 122 AJCC stage III melanoma patients who were disease-free after resection of metastatic disease in lymph nodes (15). Patients were randomized to receive five immunizations over a six-month period with either BCG alone (64 patients) or BCG with GM2 adherent to the BCG surface (58 patients). Fifty-seven patients with GM2 antibody (present naturally or vaccine-induced) had a significantly increased disease-free interval (p = .004) and overall survival (p = .02). Comparing the treatment (GM2/BCG) and control (BCG) groups, exclusion of all patients with preexisting GM2 antibodies (1 in the GM2/BCG group and 5 in the BCG group) resulted in an absolute 17% increase in disease-free survival (p = .02), and a 14% increase in overall survival at 51 months for patients receiving the GM2/BCG vaccine. However, when all patients in the two treatment groups were compared as randomized, these absolute increases were 14% for the disease-free interval and 11% for survival in the GM2/BCG treatment group, with neither result showing statistical significance. As with all previous GM2 vaccines, antibody responses were predominantly IgM, of moderate titer and short-lived with a median duration of 8–10 weeks after each immunization.

To produce higher-titered and longer-lasting IgM antibody responses against gangliosides, and to generate IgG antibodies as well, a variety of conjugate vaccines were explored (50,51). GM2 covalently attached to keyhole limpet hemocyanin (KLH) plus the immunological adjuvant QS-21 was found to be the optimal vaccine (52). KLH is a highly immunogenic protein extracted from the keyhole limpet, and it has served as a potent carrier molecule for increasing antibody responses against a variety of carbohydrate antigens. QS-21 is a potent immunological adjuvant extracted from the bark of the Quillaja saponaria tree. This conjugate vaccine induces significantly higher titer and more consistent and longer-lived IgM antibodies in melanoma patients than the GM2/BCG vaccine. In addition, for the first time, IgG antibodies were induced in most patients (52,53). Both IgM and IgG antibodies against GM2 are able to induce complement mediated lysis of GM2 positive tumor cells, and, in most cases, the IgG antibodies mediated antibody-dependent cell-mediated cytoxicity (ADCC) as well (54).

Based on these results, two randomized Phase III trials with the GM2-KLH plus QS-21 vaccine were initiated by Progenics Pharmaceuticals (Tarrytown, N.Y.) during 1996. The first is being conducted in the intergroup setting through the Eastern Cooperative Oncologic Group (ECOG), the Southwest Oncology Group, and other centers in the U.S., in melanoma patients with high-risk AJCC stage IIB or stage III melanoma who are free of disease after surgery. In this trial, patients are randomized between treatment with high-dose interferon and the GM2-KLH conjugate plus QS-21 vaccine. The second trial is being conducted in England by the Cancer Research Campaign (CRC) and the Institute of Cancer Research (ICR), with the participation of several additional hospitals in Europe and Australia. Patients with AJCC stage III melanoma who are free of disease after surgery are randomized to receive either placebo (saline) or the GM2-KLH plus QS-21 vaccine.

We have performed an immunohistological screen with a variety of monoclonal antibodies against most of the known cell surface markers of various cancers (Zhang et al., in manuscript). The gangliosides GM2, GM3, GD2, GD3, and 9-0 acetyl GD3 were the only antigens widely expressed on melanoma cells. The extensive expression of GM3 on normal tissues such as liver makes this an unlikely target for immune attack. GD3 and 9-0 acetyl GD3 have been nonimmunogenic in our initial studies with GD3/BCG, 9-0 acetyl GD3/BCG, and GD3-KLH plus QS-21 vaccines. GD2-KLH plus QS-21, however, has resulted in moderate titer IgM antibodies (median titer 1/160) in all 6 patients vaccinated. Based on this, we are initiating additional Phase I/II trials to determine optimal dose and to confirm safety after long-term immunization with a combined GM2-KLH plus GD2-KLH plus QS-21 vaccine. Phase III trials with this bivalent ganglioside vaccine will potentially follow those now being undertaken with GM2 alone in about two years, after these Phase I/II studies have been completed.

VI. CONCLUSIONS

Passively administered monoclonal antibodies (mAbs) have induced protection against experimental tumors in rodents, especially against micrometastases. Passively administered mAbs also have induced clinical responses of measurable disease in patients with melanoma or other malignancies and have induced prolonged disease-free and overall survival when administered in the adjuvant setting. Some of the antigens recognized by these mAbs are now well defined and available in purified form, making them suitable candidates for incorporation into cancer vaccines aimed at inducing long-lasting antibodies against these same antigens. The design of these vaccines and vaccine trials involves:

1. The use of well-defined purified antigens.
2. Putting these tumor antigens in close proximity to highly immunogenic nonself antigens.
3. The use of potent immunological adjuvants.
4. Vaccinating in the adjuvant setting.

Progress in the development of cancer vaccines has been dependent on the availability of surrogate markers of vaccine immunogenicity. Serological assays for quantitating vaccine-induced antibody responses are now available and being used to guide vaccine development against a number of melanoma antigens. Studies with the melanoma ganglioside GM2 are most advanced. A vaccine containing GM2-KLH conjugate plus immunological adjuvant QS-21 now induces high titers of IgM antibody against GM2 in all virtually patients and moderate-titer IgG antibodies in most patients. Natural or vaccine-induced antibodies against GM2 are associated with a significant improvement in survival in AJCC stage III melanoma patients. Randomized Phase III trials of the GM2-KLH plus QS-21 vaccine have been initiated in this country (compared to high-dose interferon) and in Europe and Australia (compared to placebo control).

REFERENCES

1. Livingston PO, and Sznol M. Vaccine therapy for melanoma. In: Balch, CM, ed. Cutaneous Melanoma, New York: JB Lippincott Company, 3rd ed., in press.

2. Fishbein DB, Robinson LE. Rabies. N Eng J Med 1993; 329: 1632–38.

3. AAP. Universal hepatitis B immunization. Pediatrics 1992; 89:795–800.

4. Rohrer JW, Rohrer SD, Barsoum A, Coggin, JH Jr. Differential recognition of murine tumor-associated oncofetal transplantation antigen and individually specific transplantation antigens by syngeneic cloned BALB/c and RFM mouse T cells. J Immunol 1994; 152:754.

5. Blachere NE, Srivastava PK. Heat shock protein-based cancer vaccines and related thoughts on immunogenicity of human tumors. Seminars Cancer Biol 1995; 6:349–355.

6. Jones PC, Sze LL, Liu PY, Morton DL, Irie RF. Prolonged survival for melanoma patients with elevated IgM antibody to oncofetal antigen. JNCI 1981; 66:249–254.

7. Livingston PO, Ritter G, Srivastava P, Padavan M, Calves MJ, Oettgen HF, Old LJ. Characterization of IgG and IgM antibodies induced in melanoma patients by immunization with purified GM2 ganglioside. Cancer Res 1989; 49:7045–7050.

8. Kawakami Y, Eliyahu S, Jennings C, Sakaguchi K, Kang X, Southwood S, Robbins PF, Sette A, Appella E, Rosenberg SA. Recognition of multiple epitopes in the human melanoma antigen gp100 by tumor-infiltrating T-lymphocytes associated with in vivo tumor regression. J Immunol 1995; 154: 3961–3968.

9. Dippold WG, Bernhard H, Peter Dienes H, Meyer zum Buschenfelde K-H. Treatment of patients with malignant melanoma by monoclonal ganglioside antibodies. Eur J Cancer Clin Oncol 1988; 24:S65–S67.

10. Houghton AN, Mintzer D, Cordon-Cardo C, Welt S, Fliegel B, Vadhan S, Carswell E, Melamed MR, Oettgen HF, Old LJ. Mouse monoclonal antibody IgG3 antibody detecting GD3 ganglioside: A phase I trial in patients with malignant melanoma. Proc Natl Acad Sci (Wash) 1985; 82:1242–1246.

11. Raymond J, Kirkwood J, Vlock D, Rabkin M, Day R, Whiteside T, Herberman R, Mascari R, Simon B. A phase 1B trial of murine monoclonal antibody R24 (anti-GD3) in metastatic melanoma (abstract). Proc Am Soc Clin Onco 1988; 7:A958.

12. Rosenberg SA, Yannelli JR, Yang JC, Topalian SL,

Schwartzentruber DJ, Weber JS, Parkinson DR, Seipp CA, Einhorn JH, White DE. Treatment of patients with metastatic melanoma with autologous tumor-infiltrating lymphocytes and interleukin 2. J Natl Cancer Inst 1994; 86: 1159–1166.

13. Schwartzentruber DJ, Hom SS, Dadmarz R, White DE, Yannelli JR, Steinberg SM, Rosenberg SA, Topalian SL. In vitro predictors of therapeutic response in melanoma patients receiving tumor-infiltrating lymphocytes and interleukin-2. J Clin Oncol 1994; 12:1475–1483.

14. Livingston PO. Approaches to augmenting the immunogenicity of melanoma gangliosides: From whole melanoma cells to ganglioside-KLH conjugate vaccines. Immunol Rev 1995; 145:147–166.

15. Livingston PO, Wong GY, Adluri S, Tao Y, Padavan M, Parente R, Hanlon C, Calves MJ, Helling F, Ritter G. Improved survival in stage II melanoma patients with GM2 antibodies; a randomized trial of adjuvant vaccination with GM2 ganglioside. J Clin Oncol 1994; 12:1036–1044.

16. Hoon DS, Yuzuki D, Hayashida M, Morton DL. Melanoma patients immunized with melanoma cell vaccine induce antibody responses to recombinant MAGE-1 antigen. J Immunol 1995; 154:73–737.

17. Mukherji B, Chakraborty NG, Yamasaki S, Okino T, Yamase H, Sporn JR, Kurtzman SK, Ergin MT, Ozols J, Meehan J. Induction of antigen-specific cytolytic T cells in situ in human melanoma by immunization with synthetic peptide-pulsed autologous antigen presenting cells. Proc Natl Aca Sci USA 1995; 92:8078–8082.

18. Krementz ET, Samuels MS, Wallace JH et al. Clinical experiences in immunotherapy of cancer. Surg Gynecol Obstet 1971; 33:209.

19. Mitchell MS, Harel W, Kempf RA, Hu E, Kan-Mitchell J, Boswell WD, Dean G, Stevenson L. Active-specific immunotherapy for melanoma. J Clin Oncol 1990; 8:856–869.

20. Morton DL, Foshag LJ, Hoon DS, Nizze JA, Famatiga E, Wanek LA, Change C, Davtyan DG, Gupta-RK, Elashoff R. Prolongation of survival in metastatic melanoma after active specific immunotherapy with a new polyvalent melanoma

vaccine. Ann Surg 1992; 216:463–482. (Erratum appears in Ann Surg 1993; 217(3):309.)

21. Berd D, Murphy G, Maguire HC, Jr. Mastrangelo MJ. Treatment of metastatic melanoma with an autologous tumor-cell vaccine: clinical and immunolgic results in 64 patients. J Clin Oncol 1990; 8:1858–1867.

22. Livingston PO, Oettgen HF, Old LJ. Specific active immunotherapy in cancer therapy, In: Mihich E, ed. Immunological Aspects of Cancer Therapeutics. John Wiley & Sons, 1982:363–404.

23. Hara I, Takechi Y, Houghton AN. Implicating a role for immune recognition of self in tumor rejection: passive immunization against the brown locus protein. J Exp Med 1995; 182:1–16.

24. Law LW, Vieira WD, Hearing VJ, Gersten DM. Further studies of the therapeutic effects of murine melanoma-specific monoclonal antibodies. Biochimica et Biophysica Acta 1994; 1226:105–109.

25. Nagy E, Berezi I, Sehon AH. Growth inhibition of murine mammary carcinoma by monoclonal IgE antibodies specific for the mammary tumor virus. Cancer Immunol Immunother 1991; 34:63–69.

26. Sugimoto Y, Watanabe M, Oh-hara T, Sato S, Isoe T, Tsuruo T. Suppression of experimental Lung Colonization of a metastatic variant of murine colon adenocarcinoma 26 by a monoclonal antibody 8F11 inhibiting tumor cell-induced platelet aggregation. Cancer Res 1991; 51:921–925.

27. Kasprzyk PG, Song SU, Di Fiore PP, King CR. Therapy of an animal model of human gastric cancer using a combination of anti-*erb*B-2 monoclonal antibodies. Cancer Res 1992; 52:2771–2776.

28. Ohnishi Y, Nakamura H, Yoshimura M, Tokuda Y, Iwasawa M, Ueyama Y. Prolonged survival of mice with human gastric cancer teated with an anti-c-ErbB-2 monoclonal antibody. Brit J Cancer 1995; 71:969–973.

29. Schreiber GJ, Hellstrom KE, Hellstrom I. An unmodified anti-carcinoma antibody, BR96, localizes to and inhibits the outgrowth of human tumors in nude mide. Cancer Res 1992; 52:3262–3266.

30. Goldstein NI, Prewett M, Zuklys K, Rockwell P, Mendelsohn

J. Biological efficacy of a chimeric antibody to the epidermal growth factor receptor in a human tumor xenograft model. Clin Cancer Res 1995; 1:1311–1318.

31. Cheung NV, Medof ME, Munn D. Immunotherapy with GD2 specific monoclonal antibodies. Advances in Neuroblastoma Res 1988; 2:619–632.

32. Hank JA, Surfus J, Gan J, Chew TL, Hong R, Tans K, Reisfeld R, Seeger RC, Reynolds CP, Bauer M, Wiersma S, Hammond D, Sondel PM. Treatment of neuroblastoma patients with antiganglioside GD2 antibody plus interleukin-2 induces antibody-dependent cellular cytotoxicity against neuroblastoma detected in vitro. J Immunotherapy 1994; 15:29–37.

33. Irie RF, Matsuki T, Morton DL. Human monoclonal antibody to ganglioside GM2 for melanoma treatment. Lancet 1989; i:786.

34. Irie RF, Morton DL: Regression of cutaneous metastatic melanoma by intralesional injection with human monoclonal antibody to ganglioside GD2. Proc Natl Acad Sci USA 1986; 83:8694–8698.

35. Dvoretsky P, Wood GS, Levy R, Warnke RA. T-lymphocyte subsets in follicular lymphomas compared with those in non-neoplastic lymph nodes and tonsils. Hum Pathol 1982; 13:618.

36. Riethmuller G, Schneider-Gadlicke E, Schlimok G, Schmiegel W, Raab R, Hoffken K, Gruber R, Pichlmaier H, Hirche H, Piehlmayr R, et al. Randomized trial of monoclonal antibody for adjuvant therapy of resected Dukes' C colorectal carcinoma. German Cancer Aid 17-1A Study Group. Lancet 1994; 343:1177–1183.

37. Baselga J, Tripathy D, Mendelsohn J, Baughman S, Benz CC, Dantis L, et al. Phase II study of weekly intravenous recombinant humanized anti-p185[her2] monoclonal antibody in patients with HER2/neu-over expressing metastatic breast cancer. J Clin Oncol 1996; 41:737–744.

38. Singhal A, Fohn M, Hakomori S-I. Induction of a α-N-acetyla-galactosamine-O-serine/threonine (Tn) antigen-mediated cellular immune response for active immunotherapy in mice. Cancer Res 1991; 51:1406–1411.

39. Fung PYS, Madej M, Koganty RR, Longenecker BM. Active specific immunotherapy of a murine mammary adenocarcinoma

using a synthetic tumor-associated glycoconjugate. Cancer Res 1990; 50:4308–4314.

40. Rose NR: Autoimmune diseases. Sci Am 1981; 244:80.

41. Bystryn JC, Ferrone S, Livingston PO, eds. Specific Immunotherapy of Cancer with Vaccines. New York: Annals of New York Academy of Sciences. 1993: Vol. 690.

42. Mittelman A, Chen ZJ, Liu CC, Hirai S, Ferrone S. Kinetics of the immune response and regression of metastatic lesions following development of humoral anti-high molecular weight-melanoma associated antigen immunity in three patients with advanced malignant melanoma immunized with mouse anti-idiotypic monoclonal antibody MK2-23. Cancer Res 1994; 54:415–421.

43. Mittelman A, Chen GZJ, Wong GY, Liu C, Hirai S, Ferrone S. Human high molecular weight-melanoma associated antigen mimicry by mouse anti-idiotypic monoclonal antibody MK2-23: modulation of the immunogenicity in patients with malignant melanoma. Clin Cancer Res 1995; 1:705–713.

44. Bystryn JC, Oratz R, Roses D, Harris M, Henn M, Lew R. Relationship between immune response to melanoma vaccine immunization and clinical outcome in stage II malignant melanoma. Cancer 1992; 69:1157–1164.

45. Miller K, Abeles G, Oratz R, Zeleniuch-Jacquotte A, Cui J, Roses DF, Harris MN, Bystryn JC. Improved survival of patients with melanoma with an antibody response to immunization to a polyvalent melanoma vaccine. Cancer 1995; 75:495–502.

46. Tsuchida T, Saxton RE, Morton DL, Irie RF. Gangliosides of human melanoma. Int J Natl Cancer Inst 1987; 78:45–54.

47. Hamilton WB, Helling F, Lloyd KO, Livingston PO. Ganglioside expression on human malignant melanoma assessed by quantitative immune thin-layer chromatography. Int J Cancer 1993; 53:566–573.

48. Tai T, Cahan LD, Tsuchida T, Saxton RE, Irie RF, Morton DL. Immunogenicity of melanoma-associated gangliosides in cancer patients. Int J Cancer 1985; 35:607.

49. Livingston PO, Natoli EJ, Calves MJ, Stockert E, Oettgen HF, Old LJ. Vaccines containing purified GM2 ganglioside elicit GM2 antibodies in melanoma patients. Proc Natl Acad Sci USA 1987; 84:2911–2915.

50. Helling F, Shang Y, Calves M, Oettgen HF, Livingston PO. Increased immunogenicity of GD3 conjugate vaccines: Comparison of various carrier proteins and selection of GD3-KLH for further testing. Cancer Res 1994; 54:197–203.

51. Livingston PO. Augmenting the immunogenicity of carbohydrate antigens. In: Livingston, PO, ed. Cancer Vaccines. Seminars in Cancer Biology, 1995, Vol. 6/6: 357–366.

52. Helling F, Zhang S, Shang A, Adluri S, Calves M, Koganty R, Longenecker BM, Yao TJ, Oettgen JF, Livingston PO. GM2-KLH conjugate vaccine: Increased immunogenicity in melanoma patients after administration with immunological adjuvant QS-21. Cancer Res 1995; 55:2783–2788.

53. Livingston PO, Adluri S, Helling F, Yao T-J, Kensil CR, Newman MJ, Marciani D: Phase I trial of immunological adjuvant QS-21 with a GM2 ganglioside-KLH conjugate vaccine in patients with malignant melanoma. Vaccine 1994; 12:1275–1280.

54. Livingston PO, Zhang S, Adluri S, Jyun YT, Walberg L, Ragupathi G, Helling F, Fleisher M. Interactions of IgG and IgM antibodies induced against GM2 ganglioside in melanoma patients by vaccination. Cancer Immunology and Immunotherapy. In press.

55. Saleh MN, Khazaeli MB, Wheeler RH, Dropcho E, Liu T, Urist M, Miller DM, Lawson S, Dixon P, Russell CH, LoBuglio AF. Phase I trial of the murine monoclonal anti-GD2 antibody 14G9a in metastatic melanoma. Cancer Res 1992; 52:4342.

7

VACCINE TRIALS IN HIGH-RISK MELANOMA
Induction of Effector T-Cell Responses to Melanoma

Walter J. Storkus, John M. Kirkwood, and Thomas Tüting
*University of Pittsburgh School of Medicine and
University of Pittsburgh Cancer Institute
Pittsburgh, Pennsylvania*

I. INTRODUCTION

Surgical resection of primary AJCC stage I/II melanoma lesions cure more than 85% of patients (1). However, those individuals with lesions > 1.5 mm in thickness or with evidence of nodal involvement remain at high risk for melanoma recurrence (1–3). These patients would be envisioned to benefit from adjunctive therapies designed to eradicate existing micrometastatic disease or to promote long-term immunity capable of preventing future melanoma progression. The clinical experience with many "classical" adjunctive therapies (chemotherapy, radiotherapy, passive antibody transfer, application of biologic response modifiers [BRM]) (4–14) have been described in detail in other chapters of this volume. (Additional strategies that may be applied as adjunctive therapies, such as gene-based therapies, have been explored largely in the setting of AJCC stage III/IV melanoma and will be described elsewhere).

The design and clinical implementation of effective immunotherapies promoting cellular immunity for the treatment of high-risk melanoma predicated upon lessons learned in the laboratory will be described in the current chapter. In the past five years, we have gained substantial mechanistic insight into cellular immune circuits that appear to be responsible for inducing and mediating the objective clinical regression of melanoma lesions in many patients undergoing immunotherapeutic treatments. Vaccines, in particular those designed to promote cellular (T cell) immunity, have now begun to assume a significant level of sophistication based, in large part, on an increasing awareness of the complex biology and intercellular dynamics of the host immune system.

II. CELLULAR IMMUNITY TO MELANOMA

For several decades, it has been generally understood that the ability of a host to reject an established tumor depends on whether a cellular antitumor immune response can be generated in that individual. In murine tumor models, the ability to confer protective antitumor immunity to naïve mice is associated with the adoptive transfer of immune lymphocytes (15–22). In contrast, the adoptive transfer of serum from immune animals to naïve mice in murine tumor models rarely provided prophylactic antitumor immunity in vivo (23,24).

In the clinical setting, several findings suggest that the immune system provides a safeguard against the development and progression of melanoma and may effectively mediate the regression of established disease. Individuals undergoing systemic immunosuppression for the maintenance of transplanted organs exhibit increased incidence of melanoma, suggesting the critical role of an intact immune system in regulating tumor progression (1,25,26). Furthermore, melanoma lesions that undergo spontaneous regression are typically infiltrated with large numbers of lymphocytes (27–33) and lymphoid infiltrates regularly characterize primary melanoma lesions. In immunotherapeutic approaches implementing tumor-based vaccines, delayed-type hypersensitivity (DTH) responses mediated principally by T lymphocytes have been observed at the site of subcutaneous or intradermal vaccine injection sites (34–36). In addition, tumor-specific cytolytic T cells have been identified in skin biopsies obtained from vaccine injection sites and from the peripheral blood of vaccinated patients (34–37). Finally, the adoptive transfer of autologous T cells expanded ex vivo from resected melanoma lesions has resulted in the objective clinical regression of residual disease (38–40).

An intriguing finding noted for many tumor histologies is the immunopathologic correlate between the degree of tumor infiltration with S100+ antigen-presenting cells (APC, i.e., dendritic cells) and reduced metastatic incidence and increased patient survival (41–44). Such APC laden with tumor-associated antigens are surmised to promote the induction and expansion of melanoma-specific T cells within tumor-draining lymphoid tissues (45–47).

III. T-CELL RECOGNITION OF MELANOMA

The mechanism by which lymphocytes, and in particular tumor-reactive T cells, recognize antigen(s) has now been largely resolved and is outlined in significant detail in a number of recent review articles (Figure 1) (18,20,33,48–50). It is now clear that T cells perceive tumor antigens as short protein fragments or peptides presented on the tumor cell surface by major histocompatibility complex (MHC) class I (present 8–12 amino acid long peptides) and class II (present somewhat longer peptides up to approximately 35 amino acids in length) molecules (49–52). These peptides may derive from any proteins synthesized by the tumor cell (i.e., proteins found in the nucleus, cytoplasm, lysosome, plasma membrane, or even secreted proteins), only a small number of which might represent "tumor-associated" or "tumor-specific." While still located within intracellular compartments, these tumor peptides associate with nascent MHC class I or class II molecules and are subsequently transported to the

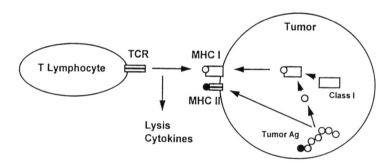

FIGURE 1 Cellular antitumor T-cell response.

cell surface, where they become accessible to T-cell scrutiny (53,54). The ability of a given peptide to bind to, and be presented by, a given MHC allele is determined by structural motifs within the peptide sequence that allow for sufficient compatibility between peptide amino acid side-chains and micropockets formed within the peptide-binding groove of the MHC molecule (33,55–58). The degree of intermolecular compatibility determines the affinity of the peptide for an individual MHC molecule, the corresponding half-life of such stable complexes, and, to a large degree, the likelihood that the peptide-MHC complex is immunogenic to the existent T-cell repertoire (59–61).

IV. MELANOMA ANTIGENS RECOGNIZED BY T CELLS

Using melanoma-reactive T lymphocytes derived from either patient peripheral blood or patient melanoma lesions as indicator reagents, multiple investigators have recently identified melanoma-associated antigens (MAA) (Table 1) (38–40,62–93). These MAA yield peptide epitopes that are recognized by T cells when presented by certain of the patient's MHC molecules. Two methodologic approaches have been implemented successfully to characterize these molecules: genetic cloning of novel melanoma-associated cDNAs and mass spectrometric analysis of peptides derived from MHC complexes expressed by tumor cells. The first, and currently the most successful approach, has been pioneered by the laboratories of Thierry Boon (Ludwig Institute, Brussels, Belgium) and Steven Rosenberg (NCI, Bethesda, MD) and involves the transfection of tumor-derived cDNA into a recipient cell line that is co-transfected with a cDNA encoding a relevant MHC class I allele. The resulting transfected cell is capable of presenting tumor antigen-derived peptides to MHC class I-restricted CTL. The ability of the transfectants to elicit the secretion of cytokine [typi-

TABLE 1
Melanoma-Associated Antigen (MAA) Epitopes Defined by HLA-Restricted T Cells

Antigen defined	Epitope sequence	HLA restriction allele	% melanoma expressing	Subcellular location	Objective clinical response	Ref.
BAGE	AARAVFLAL	Cw1601	22%	ND		69
β-catenin	SYLDSGIHF	A24	mutant	PM		80
CDK4-kinase	ACDPHSGHFV	A2	mutant	N		70
GAGE	YRPRPRRY	Cw6	24%	ND		67
gp75 (TRP-1)	MSLQRQFLR	A31		MLS	Y	68,79,148
gp100	YLEPGPVTA	A2	54%	MLS	Y	38,66,78,91, 92,147
	LLDGTATLRL	A2				
	KTWGQYWQV	A2				
	ITDQVPFSV	A2				
	VLYRYGSFSV	A2				
MAGE-1	EADPTGHSY	A1	50%	CYT	Y	37,63,84, 85,145
	SAYGEPRKL	Cw1601				

				CYT		
MAGE-3	EVDPIGHLY	A1	65–79%		Y	65,86,87,
	FLWGPRALV	A2				94,149
	MEVDPIGHLY	B44				
MART-1	AAGIGILTV	A2	90%	MLS?		61,76,83,
	ILTVILGVL	A2				90,146
MUM-1	EEKLIVVLF	B44	mutant	ND		81
NAG-V	VLPDVFIRC	A2.1	50%	GOL		93
p15	AYGLDFYIL	A24		ND	Y	82
Tyrosinase	MLLAVLYCL	A2		MLS	Y	39,40,75,
	YMDGTMSQV	A2				88,89,148
	YMNGTMSQV	A2				
	AFLPWHRLF	A24				
	SEIWRDIDF	B44				

CYT = cytoplasms; GOL = golgi; N = nucleus; PM = plasma membrane; MLS = melanosome/lysosome; ND = not determined.
Clinical trials in which complete regressions have been demonstrated upon adoptive transfer of T cells reactive with MAA or by vaccination with peptide epitopes derived from MAA are designated by Y. Mutant peptide epitopes are unique to a given patient's melanoma and are not shared by other unrelated melanoma.

cally tumor necrosis factor (TNF)-α] from melanoma-specific T cells allows for the identification of the melanoma-associated antigen (MAA) cDNA which may then be sequenced. Based on the cloned sequence of the melanoma-associated protein and the putative peptide-binding motifs identified for specific MHC alleles, a series of synthetic peptides may be generated to determine the actual peptide epitope recognized by the original CTL line or clone used in the screening process. This methodology has identified the MAA MAGE-1 (60,63,84,85), MAGE-3 (65,86,87), tyrosinase (39,40,75,77,88,89), MART-1/Melan-A (64,76,90), gp100 (38,66,91,92), tyrosinase-related protein-1 (68,79), MUM-1 (81), BAGE (69), GAGE (67), mutant cyclin-dependent kinase-4 (CDK4) (70), mutant β-catenin (80), p15 (82), and N-acetylglucosaminyltransferase V (NAG-V) (93) (see Table 1).

In the second approach, peptides are extracted from tumor cell MHC complexes by acid treatment and then analyzed by mass spectroscopy, a sensitive peptide-sequencing method capable of evaluating femtomolar concentrations of individual peptide species within complex mixtures of proteins. By sequencing, synthesizing, and screening a large number of such synthetic peptides for their ability to reconstitute T-cell recognition of lymphoid cell line targets (MHC class I matched with responder CTL) when pulsed with the synthetic peptide, naturally processed T-cell epitopes derived from gp100, tyrosinase, and MART-1 were identified (78,83,88). The consensus of currently defined MAA suggests two broad categories of antigens: melanocytic lineage differentiation antigens (MART-1/Melan-A, gp100, TRP-1, tyrosinase) and multilineage, largely tumor-restricted antigens (MAGE-1/-3, BAGE, GAGE) (73).

V. TUMOR "AUTOIMMUNITY"

An important point to be made here is that, with the exception of the mutant CDK4 and β-catenin and MUM-1 gene products identified by Wölfel et al. (70), Robbins et al. (80), and Coulie et al. (81), the other melanoma-associated antigens described above exhibit completely normal "self" germline-encoded sequences. Hence, any immune response directed against these "tumor antigens" is, by definition, an "autoimmune" response. This is a potentially important clinical consideration since the melanocytic-lineage differentiation antigens tyrosinase, gp100, TRP-1, and MART-1/Melan-A are expressed by normal dermal melanocytes as well as by the pigmented cells found in the retina (73). Theoretically, vaccine-induced immunity directed against these antigens could result in blindness (33,73,94). Fortunately, while cutaneous depigmentation (vitiligo or halo nevi) has been noted as a positive prognostic correlate of objective clinical regression in patients undergoing immunotherapy, no significant loss of visual acuity (nor any other adverse neurologic complication) has been reported to date (33,37–40,73) Genes such as MAGE-1, MAGE-3, BAGE, GAGE are not expressed in normal tissues—with the exception of testes and placenta (immunologically priviledged sites)—and their application in vaccines would not a priori be anticipated to yield pathologic autoimmunity (1–73). Clinical applications of vaccines containing MAGE-derived gene products have yielded T-cell responses in vivo in the absence of overt immunopathology (37,94), and vaccination of mice with the normal, "self" P815A antigen (expressed only by tumor cells and normal testes) produced antigen-specific CTL but no testicular pathology or infertility (73). Of note, while we and others have already identified several melanoma antigens, recent reports evaluating large numbers of melanoma-reactive T-cell clones suggest that a library of additional, novel melanoma antigens remain to be defined structurally (95). The majority of these antigens appear to be expressed by melanoma and a limited range of normal tissues including the testes, but not by normal melanocytes (95), placing them in the same category of antigens as MAGE, BAGE, and GAGE.

VI. MELANOMA VACCINE CONSTRUCTION

An effective melanoma vaccine needs to consider within its design a series of important criteria, including choice of antigen, choice of adjuvant, and choice of protocol of administration (i.e., dose, route, and schedule). These choices are selected to optimize the application of the antigen in a tissue microenvironment that favors the uptake and processing of antigen by antigen-presenting cells (APC) such as dendritic cells (DC) (45–47,96–101). The requirement for APC-processing and presentation of tumor antigens in the induction of effective antitumor reactive T cells was elegantly demonstrated by Huang et al. (101). These researchers used parent → F_1 bone-marrow chimeras to show that T-cell priming could occur only in the context of MHC products expressed by host APC rather than the MHC-peptide complexes expressed by the immunizing tumor. As we have noted above, the presence of these APC within tumors at high numbers appears to represent a positive clinical prognostic factor. By involving even larger numbers of such potent APC—either by selecting cutaneous vaccine sites distal to the tumor lesion or by ex vivo manipulation and subsequent injection of antigen-laden APC—the resulting antitumor immune response may be further enhanced (37,45,100). Potential vaccine routes of administration using APC-based approaches include subcutaneous, intravenous, or intratumoral deliveries. These considerations of adjuvant use are particularly important since melanoma vaccines may require the "breaking of functional tolerance" and limited autoimmunity against normal, "self" melanocytic lineage antigens (i.e., tyrosinase, gp100, MART-1/Melan-A, TRP-1).

The vaccine-activated or -administered DC serves as

antigen-transporting cells by trafficking to draining lymphoid tissue, principally via the afferent lymphatics (dermal injections) or peripheral blood (intravenous injection), where these APC form clusters with T cells that are themselves perfusing through the lymph node or spleen (45–47,98,100). In this microenvironment, the APC provides a series of important signals that are required for the induction, expansion, and maturation of tumor-specific T-effector cells (Figure 2): MHC + peptide (signal 1) (45,100,102), costimulation via molecules such as CD80, CD86, CD40 (100,102–104) and secreted cytokines such as IL-1, IL-12, IFN-α (105,106). Mature, antigen-specific T cells may then leave the lymphoid organs, recirculate throughout the body and, it is hoped, back to tumor lesions, where they may directly mediate the regression of established disease or recruit additional immune-cell infiltration by the paracrine elaboration of cytokines/chemokines.

Melanoma antigen for implementation in vaccines may take many forms: tumor cells (control or modified), biochemi-

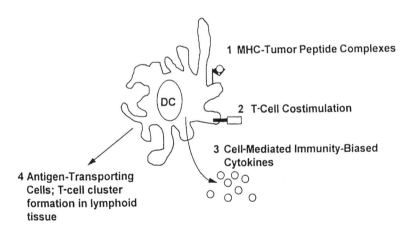

FIGURE 2 Characteristics of a vaccine stimulating an effective cellular immune response (DC + tumor antigen).

cally extracted melanoma antigens, defined synthetic peptide(s), recombinant protein, or cDNA encoding the MAA (4–8,10,36,94,107–112). Each format of MAA has its own respective benefits and disadvantages for use in vaccines (see Table 2). Crude melanoma antigen may be from an irradiated or a fixed autologous tumor, a virally or genetically modified tumor, semipurified tumor glycoproteins, tumor lysates, or acid-eluted melanoma peptides. Many current gene therapy protocols make use of cytokine gene-transfected melanomas as a therapeutic vaccine. In these protocols, it is envisioned that the genetically altered cells serve as effective antigen-presenting cells (APC) for the induction or boosting of the patient's antitumor T-cell response. Alternatively or additionally, host-effector cells (T cells, NK cells, macrophages, etc.) may be promoted to destroy the altered tumor cells, portions of which may be phagocytosed and presented in the context of MHC complexes by tissue APC within the vaccine site (101). As noted above, these epitope-laden APC may then serve as antigen-transporting cells capable of promoting T-cell induction within draining lymphoid tissues providing durable antitumor immunity.

Well-characterized melanoma antigens for implementation in vaccines may be represented by synthetic peptides derived from MAA, such as those described in Table 1 (i.e., MART-1 27–35 presented by HLA-A2.1, or MAGE-1 161–169 presented by HLA-A1). Recent data suggest that many of these peptide epitopes are capable of promoting antitumor CTL from the peripheral blood of normal donors and patients with melanoma both in vitro and in vivo (35,37,61,62, 110–112). As noted in Table 2, such MAA-derived peptides have a significant technical advantage in that they are inexpensive and biochemically well-defined entities that can be applied simply. However, they suffer the significant disadvantage that a given melanoma peptide sequence is typically presented only by a single MHC allele, which may be applied only to that subset of patients (always less than 50%; i.e.,

TABLE 2

Tumor Antigen Formats for Implementation in DC-Based Vaccines
to Elicit Antitumor T Cells

Tumor antigen format	Clinical application benefit	Clinical application disadvantage
Synthetic peptide	GMP quality peptide Easy loading of APC Selection of dominant/ subdominant epitopes	HLA restricted May lack "helper" epitopes
Recombinant protein	GMP quality protein Both MHC class I/II epitopes provided Patient HLA typing not required	Harder to access MHC class I processing pathway Less control of presentation of dominant/ subdominant Epitopes in vaccine
mRNA or cDNA	GMP quality vectors Easy application Both MHC class I/II epitopes provided Patient HLA typing not required	Harder to access MHC class II processing pathway Less control of presentation of dominant/ subdominant epitopes in vaccine

HLA-A2 is the highest frequency allele expressed by approximately 45% of humans [33]) that express that HLA allele. The patient's tumor cells should also express that specific tumor antigen, further diminishing the generic utility of a single defined peptide-based vaccine strategy. In addition, it has been hypothesized that single epitope vaccines may prove therapeutically ineffective since epitope- and/or antigen-loss tumor variants may have been immunoselected in vivo from an antigenically heterogenous population of tumor cells during the typically long periods of time associated with tumorigenesis or during active immunization (33,35,73, 113,114).

Clinical protocols using either whole tumor cells or tumor-derived peptides have demonstrated significant promise during the past decade. Objective clinical responses correlated with discernable cellular immune responses prompted by active immunization have been documented (4–6,10, 37,94). Perhaps most surprising a synthetic MAGE-3 peptide, injected subcutaneously, yielded objective clinical responses in 3 HLA-A1+ patients with melanoma, in the absence of a coinjected adjuvant (94). Such trials support the general utility of well-defined tumor peptides in the vaccine setting, as noted above, predicated on the HLA haplotypes of the patient and the documented expression of the relevant tumor antigen (from which the peptide is derived) by the patient's tumor.

While these clinical results engender significant enthusiasm, it also would be anticipated that such vaccines will further benefit from the inclusion of an MHC-presented "helper" epitope recognized by CD4+ T cells in order to optimally activate the resulting CTL response (115). Further, such epitopes may direct the generation of CD4+ cytolytic T cells or a DTH-like immune response mediated by tumor-specific CD4 + T cells within the melanoma lesion (116). These helper epitopes may either derive from MAA, such as tyrosinase (117) or they may consist of nontumor-associated peptide sequences to which CD4+ T-cell responses are readily observed in many/most individuals (118).

It is likely that additional investigation will identify CD4+ T-cell-recognized and HLA class-II-presented epitopes derived from the gp 100/pmel17, tyrosinase, and TRP-1 gene products, since each of these proteins contains a lysosomal targeting sequence (119). This places the mature protein within the intracellular compartment associated with the generation and loading of MHC class II complexes, strongly enhancing the chances for presentation of class II-associated, MAA-derived helper epitopes.

VII.   FUTURE THERAPIES

Despite some recent clinical success using "naked" peptide vaccines in melanoma patients, the full therapeutic benefit of peptide-based protocols will likely depend in significant measure upon the definition of an efficacious adjuvant, allowing for the induction and expansion of large numbers of tumor-reactive CTL in vivo. We and others (24,45,120–124) have recently demonstrated the profound biologic adjuvanticity of autologous dendritic cells in vivo in both murine tumor models and a limited series of patients with B-cell lymphoma.

Animal models have clearly documented the ability of cultured, syngeneic bone marrow-derived dendritic cells or macrophages to serve as effective immunogens of antitumor CTL in vivo when prepulsed with tumor-derived peptide epitopes (24,37,45,120,121,123). Thus, dendritic cells generated over the course of 7–8 cultures in the presence of GM-CSF and IL-4 or TNF-α could be cocultured with microgram quantities of synthetic peptides derived from proteins such as ovalbumin, HPV-16 E7, β-galactosidase, MUT1 (connexin 37), or p53, allowing for the effective loading of these peptides into DC-expressed MHC class I complexes. The subsequent vaccination and boosting of mice with as few as 10^5 of these epitope-charged cells allowed for the animals to reject a subsequent challenge with a normally lethal dose of a tumor expressing the naturally processed and presented epitope used in the vaccine (120–123). Of significant interest, in some cases, animals rejecting such a tumor challenge were also able subsequently to reject a challenge with an otherwise identical tumor that fails to express the epitope used in the original vaccination (120). These data support the concept of "epitope spreading," which may be of crucial interest in the induction of therapeutic immunity against antigenically heterogeous human lesions.

Therapeutic DC/peptide-based vaccines have also been recently evaluated (24,45,121,123), with favorable results. Thus, the majority of d5–d21-established melanomas, sarcomas, and lung carcinomas could be treated effectively, with i.v. inoculated, tumor peptide-pulsed dendritic cells. Particularly late d28 sarcomas could be induced to regress as a result of DC-based vaccination in only approximately 20% of cases (121), however, suggesting that additional intervention such as systemic cytokine administration might be applied to enhance the efficacy of such treatments.

The optimism for such DC-based applications has been augmented by recent reports in clinical studies. Of note, cultured autologous human peripheral blood APC pulsed with the MAGE-1 peptide epitopes have been shown to elicit melanoma-specific CTL within the intradermal vaccine site and in the peripheral blood of HLA-A1 patients with metastatic melanoma (37). A similar approach using freshly isolated dendritic cells (obtained by leukophoresis) pulsed with lymphoma idiotype protein has recently been implemented successfully for the treatment of patients with B-cell lymphoma (124).

Recently, we also have evaluated the impact of therapeutic tumor vaccines consisting of DC pulsed with unfractionated peptides extracted from tumor cell surface MHC class I complexes (24). This method allows for the treatment of many cancer histologies for which tumor-associated antigens have not been defined molecularly (to date) and does not require any foreknowledge of the patient's HLA typing since autologous MHC-presented peptides are applied. Freshly excised lesions are digested into single cell suspensions by enzymatic digest and subsequently washed extensively, prior to treatment with pH 3.0–3.3 acid buffer which denatures the MHC class I complexes, thus releasing tumor-associated peptides that may be recovered from the cell-free supernatant. Application of these vaccines in established murine tumor models resulted in either a profound tumor stasis period or the complete regression of tumors (24). The isolation of these heterogenous, naturally presented tumor epitopes from resected lesions may allow for the design of similar human protocols for the treatent of patients with cancer of virtually any histologic type.

Of significant current and future interest will be the application of therapies consisting of tumor-associated antigen cDNA transfected DC. Such gene-modified antigen-presenting cells will allow for a diverse series of tumor antigenic epitopes to be presented coordinately on each of the patient's MHC allelic complexes and can be applied to all patients, regardless of their HLA typing. Initial studies by Schadendorf and colleagues support the ability of human DC transfected with cDNA-encoding tyrosinase to promote antimelanoma CTL in vitro (25). Our own preliminary data support the use of DC genetically engineered for expressing tumor-associated gene products to promote the induction and expansion of anti-tumor CTL in vitro (human studies) and in vivo (in mice) (Tüting et al., unpublished results). The ex vivo expansion of highly tumor-reactive T cells derived from patient peripheral blood or lymphoid tissue using DC-based protocols for subsequent adoptive transfer into high-risk patients may also represent a tenable therapeutic option. While immunotherapies consisting of the adoptive transfer of autologous TIL or LAK cells plus IL-2 have proved effective in mediating the regression of a minority of patients with advanced metastatic melanoma (1,4,14,17,38–40,126,127), the use of DC and MAA peptide, protein, or cDNA is envisioned to yield higher frequencies of therapeutically relevant antimelanoma T cells for adoptive transfer, theoretically providing greater efficacy.

Genes encoding MAA may also be applied as therapeutic or propylactic vaccines, using alternate approaches such as "naked" DNA injection into muscle (128), recombinant viruses such as adenovirus, poxviridae, or vaccinia virus (129–131) via directed liposomes (125,132), or by bioballistic "gene gun" insertion of mRNA or cDNA into the dermis (133,134). Recently, Zhai et al. (131) protected mice against a subsequent challenge of B16 melanoma by prophylactically vaccinating them with recombinant vaccinia virus encoding the human gp100 gene product. Similarly, protective immunity to transfected tumor challenge has been demonstrated using vaccines incorporating putative tumor antigen cDNAs such as ovalbumin and β-galactosidase (135,136). Given their relative technical simplicity of clinical application, these latter approaches are attractive.

VIII. SUMMARY

The past five years have seen the rapid evolution of the molecular definition of melanoma-associated antigens (MAA). These MAA serve as logical starting points for the development of well-defined vaccines targeted for effective therapy not only for patients with established metastatic disease, but also for individuals surgically cured of disease but at high risk for recurrence. Despite the requirement that the induction of immunity against most of these MAA requires the promotion of at least limited autoimmunity, such immunotherapies appear to hold significant promise. The ideal melanoma vaccine designed to effect the systemic eradication of disseminated micrometastatic disease likely will involve the implementation of multiple MAA antigens and epitopes to circumvent immune evasion by evolving melanoma cells placed under immune selective pressure. Further, the immunogenicity of such MAA proteins/peptides most likely will be augmented significantly by the inclusion of state-of-the-art adjuvants geared toward the production of Th1-associated cellular immunity. While such approaches may be particularly salient in the context of patients with established disease whose general immunocompetency may be reduced, clearly the ideal candidates for MAA-based vaccines are those high-risk AJCC stage I/II patients treated surgically who display a high degree of immunocompetency.

The recent adoption of ex vivo antigen-loaded APC, such as cultured autologous monocytes and dendritic cells, in clinical protocols demonstrates a logical means by which to provide a relevant tumor antigen in the context of particularly immunostimulatory APC (33,37,45,137,138). Such APC may be loaded under conditions that optimize the expression of both MHC-presented tumor peptides and T-cell costimulatory molecules. Alternatively, gene therapies implementing cDNA encoding tumor antigens and/or cytokines may similarly optimize APC processing/presentation of MAA epitopes and facilitate DC-T-cell collaboration, resulting in effective induction of tumor-specific T cells in the lymphoid tissues draining the vaccination site(s). Potentiation of such antitumor effector cells might be further observed upon systemic or gene-therapy application of nontoxic doses of T-cell growth factors such as IL-2, IL-7, IL-12, or IL-15 (140–142). Additional cytokines, such as IFN-α, which appears to enhance APC function (143), facilitate CD8+ T cell induction (143), and have documented adjunctive therapeutic benefit in the melanoma setting (144) would also be attractive components in future protocol design. We are now in a favorable position to analyze the benefits of appropriately applying these recently identified tools in the context of novel adjunctive clinical trials for the treatment of patients with melanoma.

ACKNOWLEDGEMENT

The authors wish to thank Drs. Debra Ma and Cara Wilson for their critical review of this chapter. This work was supported by NIH Grant CA 157840 (WJS) and a Cancer Research Institute Clinical Investigator Award (WJS).

REFERENCES

1. Johnson TM, Smith JW, Nelson BR, Chang A. Current therapy for cutaneous melanoma. J Am Acad Derm 1995; 32:689–707.
2. Barth A, Morton DL. The role of adjuvant therapy in melanoma management. Cancer 1995; 75:726–734.
3. Mackie, RM. Strategies to reduce mortality from cutaneous malignant melanoma. Arch Derm Res 1994; 287:13–15.
4. Maeurer MJ, Storkus WJ, Kirkwood J, Lotze MT. New treatment options for patients with melanoma: Review of melanoma-derived T-cell epitope-based vaccines. Melanoma Res 1995; 5:1–14.
5. Mitchell MS, Harel W, Kempf RA, Hu E, Kan-Mitchell J, Boswell WD, Dean G, Stevenson L. Active-specific immunotherapy for melanoma. J Clin Oncol 1990; 8:856–859.
6. Wallack MK, Sivanandham M, Whooley B, Ditaranto K, Bartolucci AA. Favorable clinical responses in subsets of patients from a randomized, multi-institutional melanoma vaccine trial. Ann Surg Oncol 1996; 3:110–117.
7. Nathan PE, Mastrangelo MJ. Adjuvant therapy for cutaneous melanoma. Sem Oncol 1995; 22:647–661.
8. Livingston PO. Approaches to augmenting the immunogenicity of melanoma gangliosides: From whole melanoma cells to ganglioside-KLH conjugate vaccines. Immunol Rev 1995; 145:147–166.
9. Strom EA, Ross MI. Adjuvant radiation therapy after axillary lymphadenectomy for metastatic melanoma: Toxicity and local control. Ann Surg Oncol 1995; 2:445–449.
10. Berd D, Murphy G, McGuire HC, Mastrangelo MJ. Immunization with haptenized, autologous tumor cells induces inflammation of human melanoma metastases. Cancer 1991; 51:2731–2734.
11. Ang KK, Peters LJ, Wober RS, Morrison WH, Frankenthaler RA, Garden AS, Goefert H, Ha CS, Byers RM. Postoperative radiotherapy for cutaneous melanoma of the head and neck regions. Int J Rad Oncol Biol Phys 1994; 30:795–798.
12. Meyskens FL Jr., Liu PY, Tuthill RJ, Sondak YK, Fletcher WS, Jewell WR, Samlowski W, Balcerzak SP, Rector DJ,

Noyes RD. Randomized trial of vitamin A versus observation as adjuvant therapy in high-risk primary malignant melanoma: A Southwest Oncology Group Study. J Clin Oncol 1994; 12:2060–2065.

13. Yeung RS. Management of recurrent cutaneous melanoma. Curr Prob Cancer 1994; 18:143–186.

14. Belli F, Arienti F, Rivoltini L, Santinami M, Mascheroni L, Prada A, Ammatuna M, Marchesi E, Parmiani G, Cascinelli N. Treatment of recurrent in transit metastases from cutaneous melanoma by isolation perfusion in extracorporeal circulation with interleukin-2 and lymphokine activated killer cells. A pilot study. Mel Res 1992; 2:263–271.

15. Foley EJ. Antigenic properties of methylcholanthrene-induced tumors in mice of the strain of origin. Cancer Res 1953; 13:835.

16. Prehn RT, Main JM. Immunity to methylcholanthrene-induced sarcomas. J. Natl Cancer Inst 1957; 18:769.

17. Rosenberg SA, Spiess P, Lafreniere R. A new approach to the adoptive immunotherapy of cancer with tumor-infiltrating lymphocytes. Science 1986; 23:1318–1321.

18. Melief CJM. Tumor eradication by adoptive transfer of cytotoxic T lymphocytes. Adv Cancer Res 1992; 58:143–175.

19. Melief CJM, Kast WM. Lessons from T cell responses to virus induced tumours for cancer eradication in general. Cancer Surv 1992; 13:81–99.

20. Kast WM, Offringa R, Peters PJ, Voordouw AC, Meleon RH, van der Eb, AJ, Melief CJ. Eradication of adenovirus E1-induced tumors by E1A-specific cytotoxic T. lymphocytes. Cell 1989; 59:603–614.

21. Barth RJ Jr, Bock SN, Mule JJ, and Rosenberg SA. Unique murine tumor-associated antigens identified by tumor infiltrating lymphocytes. J Immunol 1990; 144:1531–1537.

22. Barth RJ Jr, Mule JJ, Spiess PJ, Rosenberg SA. Interferon gamma and tumor necrosis factor have a role in tumor regressions mediated by murine CD8+ tumor-infiltrating lymphocytes. J Exp Med 1991; 173:647–658.

23. Roth JA, ed. Monoclonal antibodies in Cancer. Advances in diagnosis and treatment. Mount Kisco, NY: Futura Publishing, 1986.

24. Zitvogel L, Mayordomo JI, Tjandrawan T, DeLeo AB, Clarke MR, Lotze MT, Storkus WJ. Therapy of murine tumors with tumor peptide pulsed dendritic cells: Dependence on T-cells, B7 costimulation, and Th1-associated cytokines. J Exp Med 1996; 183:87–98.

25. Penn I. Malignant melanoma in organ allograft recipients. Transplantation 1996; 61:274–278.

26. Bouwes-Bavinck JW, Hardie DR, Green A, Cutmore S, MacNaught A, O'Sullivan B, Siskind V, van der Woude FJ, Hardie IR. The risk of skin cancer in renal transplant recipients in Queensland, Australia. A follow-up study. Transplantation 1996; 61:715–721.

27. Strohal R. Immunohistological analysis of anti-melanoma host responses. Arch Dermatol Res 1994; 287:28–35.

28. Mackenson A, Carcelain G, Viel S, Raynal S, Michalaki H, Triebel F, Bosq J, Hercend T. Direct evidence to support the immunosurveillance concept in a human regressive melanoma. J Clin Invest 1994; 93:1397–1402.

29. Mihm MC Jr, Clemente CG, Cascinelli N. Tumor infiltrating lymphocytes in lymph node melanoma metastases: A histopathologic prognostic indicator and an expression of local immune response. Lab Invest 1996; 74:43–47.

30. Sensi M, Salvi S, Castelli C, Maccalli C, Mazzocchi A, Mortarini R, Nicolini G, Herlyn M, Parmiani G, Anichini A. T cell receptor (TCR) structure of autologous melanoma-reactive cytotoxic T lymphocyte (CTL) clones: Tumor-infiltrating lymphocytes overexpress in vivo the TCR-beta chain sequence used by an HLA-A2-restricted and melanocyte-lineage-specific CTL clone. J Exp Med 1993; 178:1231–1246.

31. Itoh K, Platsoucas CD, Balch CM. Autologous tumor-specific cytotoxic T-lymphocytes in the infiltrate of human metastatic melanomas. Activation by interleukin-2 and autologous tumor cells and involvement of the T-cell receptor. J Exp Med 1988; 168:1428–1434.

32. Topalian SL, Solomon D, Rosenberg SA. Tumor-specific cytolysis by lymphocytes infiltrating melanoma. J Immunol 1988; 142:3714–3725.

33. Storkus WJ, Lotze MT. Tumor antigens recognized by immune cells. In: De Vita, VT, Hellmann S, and Rosenberg, SA,

eds. Biologic Therapy of Cancer, 2nd ed. Philadelphia: JB Lippincott, 1995, 64–77.

34. Barth A, Hoon DS, Foshag LJ, Nizze JA, Famitiga E, Okun E, Morton DL. Polyvalent melanoma cell vaccine induces delayed-type hypersensitivity and in vitro cellular immune responses. Cancer Res 1994; 54:3342–3345.

35. Jager E, Ringhoffer M, Karbach J, Arand M, Oesch F, Knuth A. Inverse relationship of melanocyte differentiation antigen expression in melanoma tissues and CD8+ cytotoxic-T-cell responses: Evidence for immunoselection of antigen-loss variants in vivo. Int J Cancer 1996; 66:470–476.

36. Jaeger E, Bernhard H, Romero P, Ringhoffer M, Arand M, Karbach J, Ilsemann C, Hagedorn M, Knuth A. Generation of cytotoxic T-cell responses with synthetic peptides in vivo: Implications for tumor vaccines with melanoma-associated antigens. Int J Cancer 1996; 66:162–169.

37. Yamasaki S, Okino T, Chakraborty NG, Adkisson WO, Sampieri A, Padula, SJ, Mauri F, Muhkerji B. Presentation of synthetic peptide antigen encoded by the MAGE-1 gene by granulocyte/macrophage-colony-stimulating-factor-cultured macrophages from HLA-A1 melanoma patients. Cancer Immunol Immunother 1995; 40:268–271.

38. Kawakami Y, Eliyahu S, Delgado CH, Robbins PF, Sakaguchi K, Appella E, Yannelli JR, Adema GJ, Miki T, Rosenberg SA. Identification of a human melanoma antigen recognized by tumor infiltrating lymphocytes associated with in vivo tumor rejection. Proc Natl Acad Sci USA 1994; 91:6458–6462.

39. Robbins PF, El-Gamil M, Kawakami Y, Rosenberg SA. Recognition of tyrosinase by tumor-infiltrating lymphocytes from a patient responding to immunotherapy. Cancer Res 1994; 54:3124–3126.

40. Kang X, Kawakami Y, El-Gamil M, Wang R, Sakaguchi K, Appella E, Yanelli JR, Adema GJ, Miki T, Rosenberg SA. Identification of a tyrosinase epitope recognized by HLA-A24 restricted, tumor-infiltrating lymphocytes associated with in vivo tumor rejection. Proc Natl Acad Sci USA 1994; 91:3515–3519.

41. Furihata M, Ohtsuki Y, Sonobe H, Araki K, Ogata T, Toki T, Ogoshi S, Taniya T. Prognostic significance of simultaneous

infiltration of HLA-DR-positive dendritic cells and tumor infiltrating lymphocytes into human esophageal carcinoma. Tohoku J Exp Med 1993; 169:187–195.

42. Tsujitani S, Kukeji Y, Maehara Y, Sugimachi K, Kaibara N. Dendritic cells prevent lymph node metastasis in patient with gastric cancer. In Vivo 1993; 7:233–237.

43. Kerrebijn JD, Balm AJ, Knegt PP, Meeuwis CA, Drexhage HA. Macrophage and Dendritic Cell Infiltration in Head and Neck Squamous-Cell Carcinoma; An Immunohistochemical Study. Cancer Immunol Immunother 1994; 38:31–37.

44. Zeid NA, Muller HK. S100 Positive Dendritic Cells in Human Lung Tumors Associated with Cell Differentiation and Enhanced Survival. Pathol 1993; 25:338–343.

45. Young JW, Inaba K. Dendritic cells as adjuvants for class I major histocompatibility complex-restricted antitumor immunity. J Exp Med 1996; 183:7–11.

46. MacPherson GG, and Liu L. Dendritic cells in vivo: migration and antigen handling. Adv Exp Med Biol 1993; 329: 327–332.

47. Steinman R, Witmer-Pack M, Inaba K. Dendritic cells: antigen presentation, accessory function and clinical relevance. Adv Med Biol 1993; 329:1–9.

48. Townsend ARM. Antigen recognition by class I-restricted T lymphocytes. Ann Rev Immunol 1989; 7:601–624.

49. Townsend ARM, Rothbard J, Gotch FM, Bahadur G, Wraith D, McMichael AJ. The epitope of influenza nucleoprotein recognized by cytotoxic T lymphocytes can be defined with short synthetic peptides. Cell 1986; 44:959–968.

50. van der Bruggen P, Van den Eynde B. Molecular definition of tumor antigens recognized by T lymphocytes. Curr Opin Immunol 1992; 4:608–612.

51. Engelhard VH. Structure of peptides associated with MHC class I and class II molecules. Ann Rev Immunol 1994; 12:181–207.

52. Rammensee H-G. Chemistry of peptides associated with MHC class I and II molecules. Curr Opin Immunol 1995; 7:85–96.

53. Monaco JJ. A molecular model of MHC class I-restricted antigen processing. Immunol Today 1992; 13:173–179.

54. Cresswell P. Antigen processing. Ann Rev Immunol 1993; 11:259–293.
55. Falk K, Roetschke O, Stevanovic S, Jung G, Rammensee HG. Allele specific motifs revealed by sequencing of self peptides eluted from MHC molecules. Nature 1991; 351:290–296.
56. Kubo RT, Sette A, Grey HM, Appella E, Sakeguchi K, Zhu N-Z, Arnott D, Sherman N, Shabinowitz J, Michel H, Bodnar WM, Davis TA, Hunt DF. Definition of specific peptide motifs for four major HLA-A alleles. J Immunol 1994; 152:3913–3924.
57. Falk K, Rotzschke O. Consensus motifs and peptide ligands of MHC class I molecules. Sem Immunol 1993; 5:81–89.
58. Pamer EG, Harty JT, Bevan MJ. Precise prediction of a dominant class I MHC-restricted epitope of Listeria monocytogenes. Nature 1991; 353:852–855.
59. van der Burg AH, Visseren MJW, Brandt RMP, Kast WM, Melief CJM. Immunogenicity of peptides bound to MHC class I molecules depends on the MHC-peptide complex stability. J Immunol 1996; 156:3308–3314.
60. Sette A, Vitiello A, Reherman B, Fowler P, Nayersina R, Kast WM, Melief CJ, Oseroff C, Yuan L, Ruppert J. The relationship between class I binding affinity and immunogenicity of potential cytotoxic T cell epitopes. J Immunol 1994; 153:5586–5592.
61. van Elsas A, van der Berg SH, van der Minne CE, Borghi M, Mourer JS, Melief CJM, Schrier PI. Peptide-pulsed dendritic cells induce tumoricidal cytotoxic T lymphocytes from healthy donors against stably HLA-A 0201-binding peptides from the Melan-A/MART-1 self antigen. Eur J Immunol 1996; 26:1683–1689.
62. Celis E, Tsai V, Crimi C, DeMars R, Wentworth PA, Chesnut RW, Grey HM, Sette A, Serra HM. Induction of anti-tumor cytotoxic T lymphocytes in normal humans using primary cultures and synthetic peptide epitopes. Proc Natl Acad Sci USA 1994; 91:2105–2109.
63. van der Bruggen P, Traversan C, Chomez P, Lurquin C, De Plaen E, van den Eynde B, Knuth A, Boon T. A gene encoding an antigen recognized by cytolytic T lymphocytes on a human melanoma. Science 1991; 254:1643–1647.

64. Coulie PG, Brichard V, van Pel A, Wolfel T, Schneider J, Traversari C, Mattei S, De Plaen E, Lurquin C, Szikora JP, Boon T. A new gene coding for a differentiation antigen recognized by autologous cytolytic T lymphocytes on HLA-A2 melanomas. J Exp Med 1994; 180:35–42.

65. Gaugler B, van den Eynde B, van der Bruggen P, Romero P, Gaforio JJ, De Plaen E, Lethe B, Brasseur F, Boon T. Human gene MAGE-3 codes for an antigen recognized on a human melanoma by autologous cytolytic T lymphocytes. J Exp Med 1994; 179:921–930.

66. Bakker ABH, Schreurs MW, de Boer AJ, Kawakami Y, Rosenberg S, Adema GJ, Figdor CG. Melanocyte lineage-specific antigen gp 100 is recognized by melanoma derived tumor-infiltrating lymphocytes. J Exp Med 1994; 179:1005–1009.

67. van den Eynde B, Peeters O, De Backer O, Baugler B, Lucas S, Boon T. A new family of genes coding for an antigen recognized by autologous cytolytic T lymphocytes on a human melanoma. J Exp Med 1995; 182:689–698.

68. Wang R, Robbins PF, Kawakami Y, Kang X, Rosenberg SA. Identification of a gene encoding a melanoma tumor antigen recognized by HLA-A31-restricted tumor-infiltrating lymphocytes. J Exp Med 1995; 181:799–804.

69. Boel P, Wildmann C, Sensi ML, Brasseur R, Renauld JC, Coulie P, Boon T, van der Bruggen P. BAGE: A new gene encoding an antigen recognized on human melanomas by cytolytic T lymphocytes. Immunity 1995; 2:167–175.

70. Wolfel T, Hauer M, Schneider J, Serrano M, Wolfel C, Klehmann-Hieb E, De Plaen E, Hankeln T, Mayer zum Buschenfelde K-H, and Beach D. A p16^{INK4a}-insensitive CDK4 mutant targeted by cytolytic T lymphocytes in a human melanoma. Science 1995; 269:1281–1284.

71. Boon T, Cerrotini J-C, van den Eynde B, van der Bruggen, Van Pel A. Tumor antigens recognized by T lymphocytes. Ann Rev Immunol 1994; 12:337–365.

72. van den Eynde B, Brichard VG. New tumor antigens recognized by T cells. Curr Opin Immunol 1995; 7:674–681.

73. Boon T, van der Bruggen P. Human tumor antigens recognized by T lymphocytes. J Exp Med 1996; 183:725–729.

74. Anichini A, Maccalli C, Mortarini R, Salvi S, Mazzocchi A,

Squarcina P, Herlyn M, Parmiani G. Melanoma cells and normal melanocytes share antigens recognized by HLA-A2-restricted cytotoxic T cell clones from melanoma patients. J Exp Med 1993; 177:989–998.

75. Wolfel T, Van Pel A, Brichard V, Schneider J, Seliger B, Meyer zum Buschenfelde K-H, Boon T. Two tyrosinase non-apeptides recognized on HLA-A2 melanomas by autologous cytolytic T lymphocytes. Eur J Immunol 1994; 24:759–764.

76. Kawakami Y, Eliyahu S, Delgado CH, Robbins PF, Rivoltini L, Topalian SL, Miki T, Rosenberg SA. Cloning of the gene coding for a shared human melanoma antigen recognized by autologous T cells infiltrating into tumor. Proc Natl Acad Sci USA 1994; 91:3515–3519.

77. Brichard V, Van Pel A, Wolfel T, Wolfel C, De Plaen E, Lethe B, Coulie P, Boon T. The tyrosinase gene codes for an antigen recognized by autologous cytolytic T lymphocytes on HLA-A2 melanomas. J Exp Med 1993; 178:489–495.

78. Cox AL, Skipper J, Chien Y, Henderson RA, Darrow TL, Shabinowitz J, Engelhard VH, Hunt DF, Slingluff CL, Jr. Identification of a peptide recognized by five melanoma-specific human cytotoxic T cell lines. Science 1994; 264:716–719.

79. Wang R-F, Parkhurst MR, Kawakami Y, Robbins PF, Rosenberg SA. Utilization of an alternate open reading frame of a normal gene in generating a novel human cancer gene. J Exp Med 1996; 183:1131–1140.

80. Robbins PF, El-Gamil M, Li YF, Kawakami Y, Loftus D, Appella E, Rosenberg SA. A mutated β-catenin gene encodes a melanoma-specific angiten recognized by tumor infiltrating lymphocytes. J Exp Med 1996; 183:1185–1192.

81. Coulie PG, Lehmann F, Lethe B, Herman J, Lurquin C, Andrawiss M, Boon T. A mutated intron sequence codes for an antigenic peptide recognized by cytolytic T lymphocytes on a human melanoma. Proc Natl Acad Sci USA 1995; 92:7976–7980.

82. Robbins PF, El-Gamil M, Li YF, Topalian SL, Rivoltini L, Sakaguchi K, Appella E, Kawakami Y, Rosenberg SA. Cloning of a new gene encoding an antigen recognized by melanoma-specific HLA-A24-restricted tumor-infiltrating lymphocytes. J Immunol 1995; 154:5944–5450.

83. Castelli C, Storkus WJ, Maeurer MJ, Huang E, Pramanik B, Lotze MT. Mass spectrometric identification of a naturally-processed melanoma peptide recognized by CD8+ cytotoxic T lymphocytes. J Exp Med 1995; 181:363–366.

84. Traversai C, van der Bruggen P, Luescher IF. A nonapeptide encoded by human gene MAGE-1 is recognized on HLA-A1 by cytologic T lymphocytes directed against tumor antigen MZ2-E. J Exp Med 1992; 176:1453–1457.

85. van der Bruggen P, Szikora JP, Boel P, Wildmann C, Somville M, Sensi M, Boon T. Autologous cytolytic T lymphocytes recognize a MAGE-1 nonapeptide on melanomas expressing HLA-Cw 1601. Eur J Immunol 1994; 24:2134–2140.

86. van der Bruggen P, Bastin J, Gajeswki T, Coulie PG, Boel P, De Smet C, Traversari C, Townsend A, Boon T. A peptide encoded by human gene MAGE-3 and presented by HLA-A2 induces cytolytic T lymphocytes that recognize tumor cells expressing MAGE-3. Eur J Immunol 1994; 24:3038–3043.

87. Herman J, van der Bruggen Luescher IF, Mandruzzato S, Romero P, Thonnard J, Fleischhauer K, Boon T, Coulie PG. A peptide encoded by the human MAGE-3 gene and presented by HLA-B44 induces cytolytic T lymphocytes that recognize tumor cells expressing MAGE-3. Immunogenetics 1996; 43:377–383.

88. Skipper JCA, Hendrickson RC, Gulden PH, Brichard V, Van Pel A, Chen Y, Shabinowitz J, Wolfel T, Slingluff CL Jr., Boon T, Hunt DF, Engelhard VH. An HLA-A2-restricted tyrosinase antigen on melanoma cells results from posttranslational modification and suggests a novel pathway for processing of membrane proteins. J Exp Med 1996; 183:527–534.

89. Brichard VG, Herman J, van Pel A, Wildmann C, Gaugler B, Wolfel T, Boon T, Lethe B. A tyrosinase nonapeptide presented by HLA-B44 is recognized on a human melanoma by autologous cytolytic T lymphocytes. Eur J Immunol 1996; 26:224–230.

90. Kawakami Y, Eliyahu S, Sakaguchi K, Robbins PF, Rivoltini L, Yannelli JR, Appella E, Rosenberg SA. Identification of the immunodominant peptides of the MART-1 human melanoma antigen recognized by the majority of HLA-A2-restricted tumor infiltrating lymphocytes. J Exp Med 1994; 180:347–352.

91. Bakker AB, Schreurs MW, Tafazzul G, de Boer AJ, Kawakami Y, Adema GJ, Figdor CG. Identification of a novel peptide derived from the melanocyte-specific gp 100 antigen as the dominant epitope recognized by an HLA-A2.1-restricted anti-melanoma CTL line. Int J Cancer 1995; 62:97–102.

92. Kawakami Y, Eliyahu S, Jennings C, Sakaguchi K, Kang X, Southwood S, Robbins PF, Sette A, Appella E, Rosenberg SA. Recognition of multiple epitopes in the human melanoma antigen gp100 by tumor-infiltrating T lymphocytes associated with in vivo tumor regression. J Immunol 1995; 154: 3961–3968.

93. Guilloux Y, Lucas S, Brichard VG, Van Pel A, Viret C, De Plaen E, Brasseur F, Lethe B, Jotereau F, Boon T. A peptide recognized by human cytolytic T lymphocytes on HLA-A2 melanomas is encoded by an intron sequence of the N-acetyl-glucosaminyltransferase V gene. J Exp Med 1996; 183: 1173–1183.

94. Marchand M, Weynants P, Rankin E, Arienti F, Belli F, Parmiani G, Cascinelli N, Bourlond A, Vanwijck R, Humblet Y, Canon J-L, Laurent C, Naeyaert J-M, Plagne R, Deraemaeker R, Knuth A, Jager E, Brasseur F, Herman J, Coulie PG, Boon T. Tumor regression responses in melanoma patients treated with a peptide encoded by gene MAGE-3. Int J Cancer 1995; 63:883–885.

95. Anichini A, Mortarini R, Maccalli C, Squarcina P, Fleischhauer K, Mascheroni L, Parmiani G. Cytotoxic T cells directed to tumor antigens not expressed on normal melanocytes dominate HLA-A2.1-restricted immune repertoire to melanoma. J Immunol 1996; 156:208–217.

96. Sinkovics JG, and Horvath J. Can virus therapy of human cancer be improved by apoptosis induction? Med Hypoth 1995; 44:359–368.

97. Rankin EM. Scientific aspects of gene therapy in melanoma. Curr Opin Oncol 1995; 7:192–196.

98. Goerdt S, Kodelia V, Schmuth M, Orfanos CE, Sorg C. The mononuclear phagocyte-dendritic cell dichotomy: myths, facts, and a revised concept. Clin Exp Med 1996; 105:1–9.

99. Steinman RM, and Swanson J. The endocytic activity of dendritic cells. J Exp Med 1995; 182:283–288.

100. Stingl G, Bergstresser PR. Dendritic cells: a major story unfolds. Immunol Today 1995; 16:330–333.

101. Huang AYC, Bruce AT, Pardoll DM, Levitsky HI. Does B7.1 expression confer antigen-presenting cell capacity in tumors in vivo? J Exp Med 1996; 183:769–776.

102. Mondino A, Jenkins MK. Surface proteins involved in T cell costimulation. J Leuk Biol 1994; 55:805–815.

103. Banchereau J, Dubois B, Fayette J, Burdin N, Briere F, Miossec P, Rissoan MC, van Kooten C, Caux C. Functional CD40 antigen on B cells, dendritic cells, and fibroblasts. Adv Exp Med Biol 1995; 378:79–83.

104. Inaba K, Inaba M, Witmer-Pack M, Hatchcock K, Hodes R, Steinman RM. Expression of B7 costimulator molecules on mouse dendritic cells. Adv Exp Med Biol 1995; 378:65–70.

105. Macatonia SE, Hosken NA, Litton M, Viera P, Hsieh CS, Culpepper JA, Wysocka M, Trinchieri G, Murphy KM, O'-Garra A. Dendritic cells produce IL-12 and direct the development of Th1 cells from naive CD4+ T cells. J Immunol 1995; 154:5071–5079.

106. Zhou LJ, Tedder TF. A distinct pattern of cytokine gene expression by human CD83+ blood dendritic cells. Blood 1995; 86:3295–3301.

107. Schild H, Von Hoegen P, Schirrmacher V. Modification of tumor cells by a low dose of Newcastle disease virus II. Augmented tumor-specific T cell responses as a result of CD4+ and CD8+ T cell cooperation. Clin Immunol Immunother 1989; 28:22–29.

108. Dranoff G, Jaffee E, Lazenby A, Golumbek P, Levitsky H, Brose K, Jackson V, Hamada H, Pardoll D, Mulligan RC. Vaccination with irradiated tumor cells engineered to secrete murine granulocyte-macrophage colony-stimulating factor stimulates potent, specific, and long-lasting anti-tumor immunity. Proc Natl Acad Sci USA 1993; 90:3539–3544.

109. Hoon DS, Yuzuki D, Hayashida M, Morton DL. Melanoma patients immunized with melanoma cell vaccine induce antibody responses to recombinant MAGE-1 antigen. J Immunol 1995; 154:730–737.

110. Bakker AB, Marland G, De Boer AJ, Danen H, Adema GJ, Figdor CG. Generation of antimelanoma cytotoxic T lympho-

cytes from healthy donors after presentation of melanoma-associated antigen-derived epitopes by dendritic cells in vitro. Cancer Res 1995; 55:5330–5339.

111. Rivoltini L, Kawakami Y, Sakaguchi K, Southwood S, Sette A, Robbins PF, Marincola FM, Salgaller ML, Yannelli JR, Appella E, Rosenberg SA. Induction of tumor-reactive CTL from peripheral blood and tumor-infiltrating lymphocytes of melanoma patients by in vitro stimulation with an immunodominant peptide of the human melanoma antigen MART-1. J Immunol 1995; 154:2257–2265.

112. Salgaller ML, Afshar A, Marincola FM, Rivoltini L, Kawakami Y, Rosenberg SA. Recognition of multiple epitopes in the human melanoma antigen gp100 by peripheral blood lymphocytes stimulated in vitro with synthetic peptides. Cancer Res 1995; 55:4972–4979.

113. Maeurer MJ, Gollin SM, Storkus WJ, Swaney W, Martin DM, Castelli C, Salter RD, Knuth A, Lotze MT. Tumor escape from immune recognition I. Loss of HLA-A2 melanoma cell surface expression associated with a complex rearrangement of the short arm of chromosome 6. Clin Cancer Res 1996; 2:641–652.

114. Maeurer MJ, Gollin SM, Martin DM, Swaney W, Bryant J, Castelli C, Robbins P, Parmiani G, Storkus WJ, Lotze MT. Tumor escape from immune recognition: Lethal recurrent melanoma in a patient associated with downregulation of the peptide transporter protein TAP-1 and loss of expression of the immunodominant MART-1/Melan-A antigen. J Clin Inv 1996; in press.

115. Keene JA, Forman J. Helper activity is required for the in vivo generation of cytotoxic T lymphocytes. J Exp Med 1982; 155:768.

116. Topalian SL, MHC class II restricted tumor antigens and the role of CD4+ T cells in cancer immunotherapy. Curr Opin Immunol 1994; 6:741–745.

117. Topalian SL, Rivoltini L, Mancini M, Markus NR, Robbins PF, Kawakami Y, Rosenberg SA. Human CD4+ T cells specifically recognize a shared melanoma-associated antigen encoded by the tyrosinase gene. Proc Natl Acad Sci USA 1994; 91:9461–9565.

118. Alexander J, Sidney J, Southwood S, Ruppert J, Oseroff C, Maewal A, Snoke K, Serra HM, Kubo RT, Sette A. Development of high potency universal DR-restricted helper epitopes by modification of high affinity DR-blocking peptides. Immunity 1994; 1:751–761.

119. Vijayasaradhi S, Xu Y, Bouchard B, Houghton AN. Intracellular sorting and targeting of melanosomal membrane proteins: Identification of signals for sorting of the human brown locus protein, gp75. J Cell Biol 1995; 130:807–820.

120. Celluzzi CM, Mayordomo JI, Storkus WJ, Lotze MT, Falo LD. Peptide-pulsed dendritic cells induce antigen-specific, CTL-mediated protective tumor immunity. J Exp Med 1996; 183:283–288.

121. Mayordomo JI, Zorina T, Storkus WJ, Zitvogel L, Celluzzi C, Falo LD, Melief CJ, Ildstad ST, Kast WM, DeLeo A, Lotze MT. Bone marrow derived dendritic cells pulsed with synthetic tumour peptides elicit protective and therapeutic anti-tumor immunity. Nature Med 1995; 1:1297–1302.

122. Paglia P, Chiodoni C, Rodolfo M, and Colombo MP. Murine dendritic cells loaded in vitro with soluble protein prime CTL against tumor antigen in vivo. J Exp Med 1996; 183:317–322.

123. Mayordomo J, Loftus DJ, Sakamoto H, De Cesare CM, Appasamy PM, Lotze MT, Storkus WJ, Appella E, DeLeo AB. Therapy of murine tumors with p53 wild-type and mutant sequence peptide-based vaccines. J Exp Med 1996; 183:1357–1365.

124. Hsu FJ, Benike C, Fagnoni F, Liles TM, Czerwinski D, Taidi B, Engelman EG, Levy R. Vaccination of patients with B cell lymphoma using autologous antigen-pulsed dendritic cells. Nature Med 1996; 2:52–55.

125. Alijagic S, Moller P, Artuc M, Jurgovsky K, Czarnetzki BM, Schadendorf D. Dendritic cells generated from peripheral blood transfected with human tyrosinase induce specific T cell activation. Eur J Immunol 1995; 25:3100–3107.

126. Rosenberg SA, Packard BS, Aebersold PM, Solomon D, Topalian SL, Toy ST, Simon P, Lotze MT, Yang JC, Seipp CA. Use of tumor-infiltrating lymphocytes and interleukin-2 in the immunotherapy of patients with metastsic melanoma. New Engl J Med 1988; 319:1676–1680.

127. Gold JE, Masters TR, Osband ME. Autolymphocyte therapy. III: Effective adjuvant adoptive cellular therapy with in vivo anti-tumor specificity against murine melanoma and carcinoma using ex-vivo-activated memory T-lymphocytes. J Surg Res 1995; 59:279–286.

128. Ertl HCJ, Xhaing Z. Novel vaccine approaches. J Immunol 1996; 156:3579–3582.

129. Taylor J, Weinberg R, Taraglia J, Richardson C, Alkhatib G, Briedis D, Appel M, Norton E, Paoletti E. Non-replicating viral vectors as potential vaccines: Recombinant canary-pox virus expressing measles virus fusion (F) and hemagglutinin (HA) glycoproteins. Virology 1992; 187:321.

130. Spooner RA, Deonarian MP, Epenetos AA. DNA vaccination for cancer treatment. Gene Ther 1995; 2:173–180.

131. Zhai Y, Yang JC, Kawakami Y, Spiess P, Wadsworth SC, Cardoza LM, Couture LA, Smith AE, Rosenberg SA. Antigen-specific tumor vaccines. Development and characterization of recombinant adenoviruses encoding MART-1 or gp100 for cancer therapy. J Immunol 1996; 156:700–710.

132. Nabel GJ, Nabel EG, Yang ZY, Fox BA, Plautzz GE, Gao X, Huang L, Shu S, Gordon D, Chang AE. Direct gene transfer with DNA-liposome complexes in melanoma: expression, biologic activity, and lack of toxicity in humans. Proc Natl Acad Sci 1993; 90:11307–11311.

133. Yang N-S, Sun W-H. Gene gun and other non-viral approaches for cancer gene therapy. Nature Med 1995; 1:481–483.

134. Qui P, Zeigelhoffer P, Sun J, Yang NS. Gene gun delivery of mRNA in situ results in efficient transgene expression and genetic immunization. Gene Ther 1996; 3:262–268.

135. Chen PW, Wang M, Bronte V, Zhai Y, Rosenberg SA, Restifo NP. Therapeutic antitumor response after immunization with a recombinant adenovirus encoding a model tumor-associated antigen. J Immunol 1996; 156:224–231.

136. Ciernik IF, Berzofsky JA, Carbone D. Induction of cytotoxic T lymphocytes and antitumor immunity with DNA vaccines expressing single T-cell epitopes. J Immunol 1996; 156:2369–2375.

137. Sallusto F, Lanzavecchia A. Efficient Presentation of Soluble

Antigen by Cultured Human Dendritic Cells is Maintained by Granulocyte/Macrophage Colony-Stimulating Factor Plus Interleukin 4 and Downregulated by Tumor Necrosis Factor Alpha. J Exp Med 1994; 179:1109–1118.

138. Bernhard H, Disis ML, Heimfeld S, Hand S, Gralow JR, Cheever MA. Generation of immunostimulatory dendritic cells from human CD34+ hematopoietic progenitor cells of the bone marrow and peripheral blood. Cancer Res 1995; 55:1099–1104.

139. Xhaing Z, Ertl HCJ. Manipulation of the immune response to a plasmid-encoded viral antigen by coinoculation with plasmids expressing cytokines. Immunity 1995; 2:129–135.

140. Rao JB, Chamberlain RS, Bronte V, Caroll MW, Irvine KR, Moss B, Rosenberg SA, Restifo NP. IL-12 is an effective adjuvant to recombinant vaccinia virus-based tumor vaccines. J Immunol 1996; 156:3357–3365.

141. Irvine KR, Rao RB, Rosenberg SA, Restifo NP. Cytokine enhancement of DNA immunization leads to effective treatment of established pulmonary metastases. J Immunol 1996; 156:238–245.

142. Zitvogel L, Couderc B, Mayordomo JI, Robbins PD, Lotze MT, Storkus WJ. IL-12 engineered dendritic cells serve as effective tumor vaccine adjuvants in vivo. An. NY Acad Sci 1996; in press.

143. Belardelli F, Gresser I. The neglected role of type I interferon in the T-cell response: Implications for its clinical use. Immunol Today 1996; 17:369–372.

144. Kirkwood JM, Strawderman MH, Ernstoff MS, Smith TJ, Borden EC, Blum RH. Interferon alpha-2b adjuvant therapy of high-risk resected cutaneous melanoma: The Eastern Cooperative Oncology Group Trial EST 1684. J Clin Oncol 1996; 14:7–17.

145. Schultz-Thater E, Juretic A, Dellabona P, Luscher U, Siegrist W, Harder F, Heberer M, Zuber M, Spagnoli GC. MAGE-1 gene product is a cytoplasmic protein. Int J Cancer 1994; 59:435–439.

146. Kawakami Y, Eliyahu S, Sakaguchi K, Robbins PF, Rivoltini L, Yannelli JR, Appella E, Rosenberg SA. Identification of the immunodominant peptides of the MART-1 human melanoma

antigen recognized by the majority of HLA-A2-restricted tumor infiltrating lymphocytes. J Exp Med 1994; 180:347–352.

147. Taajes DJ, Arendash-Durand B, von Turkovich M, Trainer TD. HMB-45 antibody demonstrates melanosome specificity by immunoelectron microscopy. Arch Pathol Lab Med 1993; 117:264–268.

148. Horikawa T, Norris DA, Johnson TW, Zekman T, Dunscomb N, Bennion SD, Jackson RL, Morelli JG. DOPA-negative melanocytes in the outer root sheath of human hair follicles express premelanosomal antigens but not a melanosomal antigen or the melanosome-associated glycoproteins tyrosinase, TRP-1, or TRP-2. J Inv Dermatol 1996; 106:28–35.

149. Kocher T, Schultz-Thater E, Gudat F, Schaefer C, Casorati G, Juretic A, Willimann T, Harder F, Herberer M, Spagnoli GC. Identification and intracellular location of MAGE-3 gene product. Cancer Res 1995; 55:2236–2239.

8

ADJUVANT CHEMOTHERAPY FOR MALIGNANT MELANOMA

Agop Y. Bedikian and Sewa Singh Legha
The University of Texas M.D. Anderson Cancer Center
Houston, Texas

I. INTRODUCTION

Malignant melanoma arising from the skin and mucous membranes occurred in an estimated 34,100 individuals in the U.S. in 1995. Currently responsible for approximately 7,000 deaths per year, mortality from melanoma is rising, although less rapidly than the incidence of the disease.

The treatment of choice for melanoma that is localized to its primary site of origin in the skin is wide local excision.

This procedure controls the disease in 70–80% of the patients. The risk of tumor recurrence is related primarily to tumor thickness. In patients with thin primaries <0.75 mm in Breslow depth, the 5-year survival rate is greater than 95%. In patients with tumor thickness >4 mm, it is 50% (1). The regional lymph nodes are the initial site of metastasis following surgical removal of the primary in more than 50% of patients. Patients with melanoma metastatic to regional lymph nodes (stage III) have a poor prognosis, with a risk of relapse exceeding 60–70% over a period of 5 to 10 years following lymph node dissection. The median survival of melanoma patients with regional lymph node metastases is 2 years; the median time to relapse is 12 months, with a range of 9–18 months (2,3). Trials of adjuvant chemotherapy and chemoimmunotherapy have been directed toward these patients in an effort to increase their survival since both therapies have been found to be more effective with small tumor mass (4).

II. SYSTEMIC THERAPY TRIALS

Postoperative adjuvant systemic chemotherapy has been widely tested during the past 20 years (5). Chemotherapy trials in patients with metastatic melanoma showed that dacarbazine (DTIC)® has consistent efficacy against metastatic malignant melanoma, with an overall single agent activity rate of 20% (6). The other classes of drugs with rates of objective antitumor activity between 10% and 15% are the nitrosoureas, vinca alkaloids, and platinum compounds (7); these are reviewed elsewhere in this volume. These antineoplastic agents, alone and in multidrug combinations, were therefore evaluated in adjuvant treatment protocols. The initial adjuvant chemotherapy trials reported survival benefit compared with historical controls (8,9). To confirm this, several prospective randomized chemotherapy and chemoimmunotherapy trials were conducted. The findings, as summarized in Tables 1 and 2, are the subject of this review.

The results of diverse adjuvant trials using only interferons or vaccines of several categories as immune response modifiers are reviewed elsewhere in this volume.

A. Systemic Chemotherapy Trials

A Phase III prospective trial involving 117 randomly assigned patients with Clark's level III–V primary melanoma

TABLE 1
Results of Adjuvant Chemotherapy Trials

Study	AJCC-UICC stage	Number of patients	Randomized treatment group	Results
Banzet et al. (10)	I,II	117	VLB/TP/ MTX/P/ STR Control	No difference in DFS overall; DFS of treated males was better (81% vs. 65% at 2 yr, p < 0.05)
Hill et al. (11)	I,II,III	174	D Control	Adverse impact of D on DFS (28% vs. 45% at 2 yr)
Tranum et al. (12)	I,II	123	B/HU/D Control	No difference
Karakousis and Emrich (13)	III,IV	135	B/AD/VCR Control	DFS of treated group was better (38% vs. 24% at 2 yr, p = 0.034); no survival difference

Abbreviations: VLB = vinblastine, TP = thiotepa, MTX = methotrexate, P = procarbazine, STR = streptonigrin, D = dacarbazine, B = carmustine, HU = hydroxyurea, AD = dactinomycin, VCR = vincristine, DFS = disease-free survival, OS = overall survival.

TABLE 2

Results of Adjuvant Chemoimmunotherapy Trials

Study	AJCC-UICC stage	Number of patients	Treatment group	Results
Jacquillat et al. (25)	I,II	67 men	D/VLB/TP/MTX/P/STR D/VLB/TP/MTX/P/STR/BCG/CP	No difference
		82 women	D/VLB/TP/MTX/P/STR Control	DFS was in favor of women given therapy (p < 0.05)
Wood et al. (26,27)	II,III	69	D BCG D/BCG	OS with combined R_x was better than D (p < 0.01) and BCG (p < 0.05)
Terry et al. (28)	II,III	181	MeCCNU BCG BCG/TCV Control	No difference
Quagliana et al. (29)	III,IV	161	B/HU/D B/HU/D/BCG	B/HU/D was superior in DFS (p = 0.057) and OS (p = 0.007)

Study	Stage	N	Treatment	Result
Cunningham et al. (30)	I,II	471	BCG Control	No difference
	III	181	BCG	No difference
Quirt et al. (31,32)	II,III IV	94	D/BCG D/BCG Control	DFS and OS was better with D/BCG but not significantly
Veronesi et al. (33)	II,III	761	D BCG D/BCG Control	No difference
Balch et al. (34)	III,IV	113	D/CTX/CP CP	No difference
Sterchi et al. (35)	I,II,III	70	D D/MER D/ESTRACYT	No difference
Karakousis and Emrich (36)	II,III	82	BCG Control	No difference

Abbreviations: D = dacarbazine, VLB = vinblastine, TP = thiotepa, MTX = methotrexate, P = procarbazine, STR = streptonigrin, BCG = bacillus Calmette-Guerin, CP = Corynebacterium parvum, TCV = tumor cell vaccine, B = carmustine, HU = hydroxyurea, CTX = cyclophosphamide, MER = methanol-extractable residue, L = lomustine, DFS = disease-free survival, OS = overall survival.

was first reported by Banzet et al. (10). Sixty-two received postoperative chemotherapy (15 patients with limb primary also received intra-arterial dacarbazine and vincristine), and 55 underwent surgery only. Systemic chemotherapy consisted of a combination of procarbazine, vinblastine, thiotepa, streptonigrin, and methotrexate. At a short median follow-up of 19 months, recurrences occurred in 35% of the control group and in 16% of the chemotherapy group overall (p < 0.05). The difference between the disease-free survival of treated and control groups was significant only for men, where 81% of the treated subjects were disease-free compared with 65% of the control group at a follow-up of 2 years (p < 0.05).

The Central Oncology Group (COG) (11) conducted a randomized trial in 174 patients with primary melanoma or melanoma metastatic to regional lymph nodes rendered free of disease surgically. Half received dacarbazine at 4.5 mg/kg/day for 10 days for 4 courses in one year, and the other half formed the control group. At a median follow-up of 2.5 years, the control group demonstrated significantly better disease-free survival (45%) than did the dacarbazine-treated group (28%). The overall survival rate of the control group was superior as well. The prognostic factors evaluated between the two groups were comparable, and the apparent detrimental effect of chemotherapy could not be explained by problems in randomization.

The Southwest Oncology Group (SWOG) conducted a study in 123 patients with localized, clinical stage I (Clark level III or more) following surgical resection of primary melanoma (12). Fifty patients were randomly assigned to a combination chemotherapy regimen containing carmustine (150 mg/m² every 8 weeks), hydroxyurea (1500 mg/m³/day × 5 every 4 weeks), and dacarbazine (150 mg/m²/day × 5 every 4 weeks) for one year. The control group was followed without any treatment. The median disease-free survival for the treated group was 6 years, compared with 7.1 years for the control group. Both groups experienced identical survival: 65% at 6 years.

Karakousis and Emrich, of the Roswell Park Memorial

Institute, reported on another study involving 135 patients with regional or distant metastatic melanoma who underwent resection of the recurrent tumor (13). They were randomly assigned either to a chemotherapy group (70 patients) or to an observation group (65 patients). The chemotherapy included carmustine (80 mg/m^2) every 4 weeks and both actinomycin-D (0.01 mg/kg) and vincristine (1.0 mg/m^2) every 2 weeks for a total of 6 months. At a median follow-up of 33 months, relapses were observed in 72% of the patients in the observation group compared with 58% of the patients who received therapy (p = 0.021). At 2 years, the proportion of patients free of disease was significantly higher in the chemotherapy group (38%) than in the control group (24%), (p = 0.034), although no survival impact of this difference was demonstrated.

Overall, these data with adjuvant chemotherapy in melanoma are largely negative but with several caveats. Most of the studies done to date were conducted either with single-agent chemotherapy or with combinations of drugs which in general may have represented poor choices of drugs in terms of their efficacy against metastatic melanoma. These trials encompassed very heterogenous patient populations with markedly different risks of relapse. Before we can categorically exclude a benefit from chemotherapy in adjuvant therapy of high-risk melanoma, it may be argued that more modern regimens of combination chemotherapy containing at least dacarbazine, cisplatin, and either vinblastine or BCNU need to be tested. In the current situation, when the impact of polychemotherapy with regimens such as BCNU-cisplatin-dacarbazine and tamoxifen (the "Dartmouth" combination) has yet to be established as superior to dacarbazine alone, it may also be prudent to await the results of such intergroup trials (ECOG/M 91–140). One would also limit the initial studies to AJCC stage III patients, due to their more consistently elevated risk of relapse. Stage II patients should not be included unless the results are sound and positive in stage III, since their lower and later risk profile requires greater numbers and longer intervals of assessment to be informative.

B. Systemic Chemoimmunotherapy Trials

1. *Microbial Immunostimulants BCG and C. Parvum*

Since the observation of objective tumor regression of human melanoma with bacillus Calmette-Guerin (BCG) administered intradermally by Morton et al. in the late 1960s (14), numerous studies have been initiated to delineate the role of microbial immunostimulants, including BCG and C. parvum in the adjuvant therapy of melanoma. Based on the observation of survival benefit from BCG in nonrandomized studies, 5 randomized studies were undertaken to compare adjuvant BCG with observation in stages I–III melanoma patients rendered free of disease surgically (15–19). The largest study was conducted by the Eastern Cooperative Oncology Group (ECOG) and reported by Cunningham et al. (15). In this study, 474 patients with primary or regional lymph node metastases were randomized to receive immunotherapy with Tice strain BCG (18 months) or no further therapy. The results of this and all subsequent large multicenter randomized studies of microbial immunostimulants showed no statistically significant benefit with BCG in disease-free and overall survival. Similarly, three randomized adjuvant studies (20–22) compared C. parvum therapy with observation, and two compared it to BCG (23,24), in patients who had resection of the primary tumor or in-transit or lymph node metastases. No significant improvement in disease-free and/or overall survival was observed.

In a trial complimentary to an earlier study of chemotherapy (10), Jacquillat et al. treated 149 patients with Clark level III–V melanoma (25). Sixty-seven men were randomly assigned into one of two treatment groups: chemotherapy that utilized dacarbazine (300 mg/m^2) together with procarbazine, vinblastine, thiotepa, streptonigrin, and methotrexate; or chemoimmunotherapy utilizing the same chemotherapy in combination with BCG and C. parvum. Eighty-two women were assigned randomly to either the control group (43 women) or to a chemoimmunotherapy group (39 women) that received the same chemoimmunotherapy as the men's group. The relapse-free survival of the men showed no significant difference between the treatment groups (see Table 2). In women, however, there was a significantly lower relapse rate with chemoimmunotherapy (3%) as compared with surgery alone (16%).

Wood et al. reported a controlled study conducted at Massachusetts General Hospital which randomly assigned 27 patients with primary melanoma, Breslow thickness >1.5 mm, and 42 patients with regional lymph node metastasis to one of three therapies: 1) immunotherapy with BCG; 2) chemotherapy with dacarbazine 200 mg/m²/day × 3 days a month for 6 months, then every 2 months for 6 months, then every 3 months during the second year; or 3) chemoimmunotherapy with both BCG and dacarbazine (26,27). No difference in disease-free survival was found among the three treatment groups. However, the overall survival of the group treated with chemoimmunotherapy was significantly superior to the other modalities of treatment in an initial report. The findings were the same if the comparison was limited to patients with regional lymph node metastasis only, or to these patients taken together with patients without regional lymph node metastasis. The group using dacarbazine alone was discontinued due to the early appearance of an inferior survival rate.

In 1975, the National Cancer Institute began a clinical trial to evaluate the efficacy of chemotherapy and immunotherapy in 181 patients with elevated risk for melanoma recurrence (28). The patients underwent wide excision of their melanoma and dissection of the regional lymph nodes. They were then randomly assigned to receive either methyl-CCNU, BCG, BCG plus allogeneic cultured melanoma cells, or no further treatment. The results of the study were reported by Terry et al. in 1982, showing that neither of the two immunotherapy treatments nor the methyl-CCNU treatment had significantly improved the disease-free or overall survival when compared with surgery only.

SWOG treated 86 patients with carmustine, hydroxyurea, and dacarbazine (BHD regimen) and 75 patients with BHD plus BCG immunotherapy in a randomized clinical trial, starting within a month after complete resection of regional metastatic or solitary distant metastatic disease (29). The results of the study were reported in abstract form by Quagliana et al. in 1980. There was no difference in relapse rates among the treatment groups. The disease-free interval and overall survival, however, favored chemotherapy alone.

The ECOG Trial E1673 studied the effect of adjuvant BCG and dacarbazine on disease recurrence and survival (30). After surgery, 474 patients with primary melanoma and 181 patients with in-transit or regional lymph node metastases were randomly assigned to the respective study groups. Adjuvant treatment with BCG was compared with observation for patients with primary melanoma but no regional disease, while results with BCG were compared to those with dacarbazine plus BCG in patients with regional metastases. The results of the study were reported preliminarily by Cunningham et al., showing no significant differences in relapse-free or overall survival among the treatment groups and the control arm.

The NCI–Canada Clinical Trials Group studied the effects of chemoimmunotherapy in patients with Clark's levels III–V melanoma, in-transit or lymph node metastases randomly assigned to either observation or therapy after appropriate surgery (31,32). The chemoimmunotherapy group received dacarbazine (850 mg/m^2/day) every 4 weeks × 2 courses plus BCG (intradermally every 2 weeks) for 2 years. As reported by Quirt et al., at a median follow-up of 43 months (minimum 22 months), the relapse-free and overall survival rates favored the treated group, but the difference was not statistically significant (p > 0.1). Routine use of this adjuvant treatment was not recommended.

The World Health Organization (WHO) conducted a large multi-institutional trial in 761 high-risk melanoma patients with either histologically confirmed regional lymph node metastasis (pathological stage III) or Clark's level III–V cutaneous melanoma of the trunk with uninvolved regional nodes (pathological stage II)(33). The patients were assigned randomly to one of four groups: 1) surgery alone (185 patients); 2) surgery followed by dacarbazine at 200 mg/m^2/day × 5 every 4 weeks (192 patients); 3) surgery followed by BCG, (203 patients); or 4) surgery followed by both dacarbazine and BCG, (181 patients). In 1982, Veronesi et al. reported that over 70% of the patients had experienced tumor relapse. No significant difference in relapse-free or overall survival was demonstrated among the four groups.

The Southeastern Cancer Study Group reported the effects of C. parvum in a trial including 82 patients with advanced regional metastases and 31 with isolated distant metastases randomly assigned after resection either to immunotherapy with C. parvum alone or to chemotherapy including dacarbazine and cyclophosphamide (both at 600 mg/m^2 every 3 weeks) (34). Balch et al. reported no significant difference in disease-free survival between the groups. The use of systemic chemotherapy had no therapeutic effect in this high-risk patient population with melanoma.

Another study of chemoimmunotherapy was conducted by Sterchi et al. in North Carolina, enrolling 70 patients with melanoma of Clark's level II–V or with regional lymph node or in-transit metastases. Patients were randomly assigned to either dacarbazine alone at 300 mg/m^2/day × 5 days every 35 days for 2 years or dacarbazine plus methanol extracted residue (MER) of BCG intradermally every 35 days for one year (35). Neither regimen provided an advantage in disease-free or overall survival independent of clinical stage of the disease.

The Karakousis at Roswell Park Memorial Institute evaluated BCG vs. Estracyt® and dacarbazine in 57 patients with stage I and 25 patients with stage II melanoma randomly assigned to receive intradermal BCG vs. dacarbazine at 200 mg/m²/day × 5 days every 4 weeks plus Estracyt at 15 mg/kg by mouth vs. observation for one year. At a median follow-up of 73 months, 38% of the patients had relapsed with neither a disease-free nor an overall survival benefit for one or the other treatment group (36).

Group Inter-France initiated a trial of adjuvant treatment of patients with either Clark's level III, IV, or V melanoma, or with positive regional lymph nodes in 1975 (37). After surgical removal of all detectable disease, the patients were randomly assigned to either BCG for 2 years or adjuvant chemotherapy combining dacarbazine, Lomustine, and VM26 for 6 months followed by BCG. Of the 284 patients, 136 were assigned to the immunotherapy group and 148 to the chemoimmunotherapy group. In 1984, at a median follow-up of 3 years, Misset et al. reported that there was no difference among the groups in regard to disease-free survival, but despite this, a significant difference in overall survival was noted in favor of immunotherapy alone (p = 0.03).

2. *Levamisole*

Following the demonstration of the antitumor activity of levamisole and its effects on the T cells, polymorphonuclear leukocytes, monocytes, and macrophages, and the reports of its beneficial effects in the treatment of cancer of the breast and the lung, the European Organization for Research on Treatment of Cancer (EORTC) evaluated its role in operable melanoma. More than 200 patients with surgically resected melanoma of Clark levels III or greater, Breslow thickness >1.5 mm, were randomly assigned to one of three groups

(38). Patients received either adjuvant dacarbazine (250 mg/m²/day × 5 days, monthly for 6 months), levamisole, or placebo. No significant difference was noted in overall survival or disease-free survival among the three groups, as reported by Czarnetzki et al.

In 1976, the EORTC Melanoma Group embarked upon an adjuvant study (EORTC Protocol 18761) to compare the value of dacarbazine and levamisole in reference to placebo for the treatment of high-risk stage I patients. The final analysis included 274 patients (39). Seventy-seven patients received dacarbazine at 250 mg/m²/day × 5 days every 28 days, 101 patients received levamisole at 150–250 mg/day × 2 days weekly for 2 years; and 96 patients received placebo. After a mean follow-up time of 3 years, no significant difference was noted among the three groups in terms of disease-free or overall survival.

Similarly, Spitler and Sagebiel conducted a randomized double-blind trial of levamisole versus placebo as adjuvant therapy for surgical treatment of melanoma. One hundred four patients received levamisole and 99 received placebo. The preliminary analysis and reanalysis after long-term follow-up (median = 10.5 years) showed that there was no difference between the treatment and the control groups with regard to disease-free interval, time to appearance of visceral metastases, or survival (40).

In contrast, the National Cancer Institute of Canada conducted a Phase III study in 543 patients with completely resected intermediate- or high-risk melanoma randomized to one of 4 study groups; 1) levamisole on 2 consecutive days weekly for 3 years; 2) BCG for 3 years; 3) BCG alternating with levamisole every 8 weeks for 3 years; or 4) observation. At median follow-up of 8.5 years, there was a 29% reduction in mortality and recurrence rates in patients treated with levamisole alone, as compared with the observation group, (p = 0.08 and 0.09 respectively). The degree of improvement in survival rate and tumor recurrence rate in patients treated with BCG alone or with levamisole alternating with BCG was only marginal (41). These results suggest a need for further investigation of the usefulness of levamisole as adjuvant treatment in patients with melanoma.

Overall, the results of nonspecific immunotherapy used alone or in combination with chemotherapy are negative. However, the chemotherapy used in many of these trials was not sufficiently active to give optimal results. Consequently, additional studies with more intense combination chemotherapy regimens are warranted and should be carried out in a controlled randomized fashion.

III.   REGIONAL CHEMOTHERAPY

The experience with adjuvant regional chemotherapy for the prevention of tumor recurrence in high-risk patients with melanoma of the extremities is limited. The results of several studies indicate a beneficial effect of perfusion as an adjuvant treatment based on comparison with historical controls; these have been summarized by Cumberlin et al. (42). In a recent study reported by Baas et al., isolated hyperthermic regional perfusion including melphalan with or without dacarbazine was used in 22 patients with subungual melanoma (43). Eleven patients had an advanced primary alone, 11 patients also had in-transit metastasis, satellitosis, or regional lymph node metastases. All patients had primaries with a Breslow thickness of >1.5 mm. Melphalan in dosages 1–1.5 mg/kg for the lower extremity and 0.5–0.7 mg/kg for the upper extremity was given after primary surgical therapy. With a minimum follow-up of 4.5 years, 55% of the patients developed distant metastases, including 36% of the patients with primary melanoma only. Median survival of all patients was 3 years, and the overall 5-year survival rate was 40%.

In Rhode Island, between 1962 and 1979, Rege et al.

treated 39 patients who had clinical stage I melanoma of the extremities with hyperthermic isolated limb perfusion using melphalan in conjunction with wide local resection with split-thickness skin graft and regional lymphadenectomy (44). The results of this study were compared with those from a control group of 75 patients with clinical stage I extremity melanoma; these patients were treated by conventional methods including local excision and wide local excision with or without regional lymph node dissection. The patients in the perfusion group and the control groups were similar in pretreatment characteristics, except that the control group had more favorable tumor location and lower Clark level of invasion. The perfusion treatment group had significantly longer disease-free and overall survival. Three patients in the perfusion group failed loco-regionally, and 5 patients developed distant metastases. In the control group, there were 17 loco-regional failures, and 7 patients developed distant metastases. The loco-regional failure rate was reduced by perfusion (p = 0.04, Fisher exact test).

In a similar retrospective study, Franklin et al. reported on a 20-years experience in which 227 perfused stage I melanoma patients from Groningen were compared with 238 matched controls from 5 hospitals in the Netherlands and Westphalia (45). All patients underwent excision of primary melanoma of 1.5 mm or greater Breslow thickness. With corrections for tumor thickness, it was not possible to demonstrate a statistically significant beneficial effect for perfusion in terms of time to limb-tumor recurrence, time to lymph node recurrence, time to distant metastasis, disease-free interval, or survival. This group recommended that adjuvant isolated perfusion should only be performed in the framework of a phase III trial for adjuvant therapy of stage I (localized) melanoma.

In a prospective randomized study of 107 patients with melanoma of the extremities, Ghussen et al. treated 54 patients with only wide excision and regional lymph node dissection; 53 others received hyperthermic perfusion with melphalan at 1.0 mg/kg for the upper extremity and 1.5 mg/kg for the lower extremity in addition (46). An interim evaluation of the control group showed that there were 7 recurrences in stage I, 7 in stage II, and 12 in stage III. In the melphalan-perfused group there was one relapse in stage I, one in stage II, and 4 in stage III. These results are significant for stage I and II (p = 0.05) and for stage III (p = 0.01), suggesting benefit from hyperthermic perfusion. Further, there was statistically-significant advantage favoring the perfusion group both for disease-free and for overall survival. The trial was closed prematurely (with smaller numbers of patients and shorter follow-up). Definitive conclusions regarding the efficacy of the adjuvant perfusion cannot be drawn from this trial.

The Swedish Melanoma Study Group conducted a prospective randomized trial testing regional hyperthermic perfusion with melphalan after surgery for recurrent melanoma of the extremities (47). Sixty-nine patients with recurrent melanoma were allocated randomly to surgery (36 patients) or surgery plus regional perfusion (33 patients). Prognostic variables were evenly distributed in the groups. Hafstrom et al. reported that there was a significant improvement in tumor-free survival (p = 0.044) in favor of the perfusion group. The overall survival of the perfused group was better than that of the controls, but the difference did not reach statistical significance.

IV. CONCLUSION

The main objective of adjuvant chemotherapy in high-risk melanoma patients is to eradicate occult micrometastases in an effort to prevent relapse and to improve survival. Based on the results of published data, three general conclusions can be drawn. First, dacarbazine, the most active single agent in advanced melanoma, has been most widely evaluated in adjuvant settings, primarily as a single agent but also in multidrug combinations. To date, the results have revealed no consistent or significant impact on survival. Because the chemotherapy regimens used in the trials reviewed in this chapter were generally associated with low response rates (<30%) which usually were of short duration when tested against advanced disease, their lack of a significant impact on tumor recurrence and survival in the adjuvant setting is not surprising. The efficacy of more modern combination chemotherapy regimens of higher activity in advanced disease needs to be tested before discarding the possibility of benefit from adjuvant chemotherapy. Second, regional isolated limb perfusion with melphalan, with a response rate of 30–70% in patients with loco-regional melanoma involving an extremity, has been inadequately represented in randomized adjuvant clinical trials, although a multicenter study of the North American Perfusion Group and WHO/EORTC is recently concluded. Third, the roles of both the recently established intense biochemotherapy regimens and isolated hyperthermic perfusion therapy with melphalan in combination with tumor necrosis factor need further investigation in the adjuvant setting.

REFERENCES

1. Balch CM, Soong S-G, Shaw HM, et al. An analysis of prognostic factors in 8500 patients with cutaneous melanoma. In Cutaneous melanoma, 2nd ed. (C.M. Balch, A.N. Houghton, G.W. Milton, et al. eds.). Philadelphia: J.B. Lippincott, 1992:165.
2. Cascinelli N, Vaglini M, Nava M, et al. Prognosis of skin melanoma with regional node metastases (Stage II). J Surg Oncol 1984; 25:240.
3. Singletary SE, Shallenberger R, Guinee VF, McBride CM. Melanoma with metastasis to regional axillary or inguinal lymph nodes: Prognostic factors and results of surgical treatment in 714 patients. South Med J 1988; 81:5.

4. Veronesi U, Adamus J, Aubert C, et al. A randomized trial of adjuvant chemotherapy and immunotherapy in cutaneous melanoma. N Eng J Med 1982; 307:913.

5. Balch CM, Hersey P. Current status of adjuvant therapy. In: Cutaneous melanoma (C.M. Balch & G.W. Milton, eds.). Philadelphia: J.B. Lippincott, 1985:197.

6. Luce JK, Thurman WG, Isaacs BL, et al. Clinical trials with the antitumor agent 5-(3,3-dimethyl-1-triazeno)imidazole-4-carboxamide (NSC-45388) Cancer Chemo Rep Part I. 1970; 54:119.

7. Luce JK. Chemotherapy of malignant melanoma. Cancer 1972; 30:1604.

8. Gutterman JU, Mavligit GM, Gottlieb JA, et al. Chemoimmunotherapy of disseminated malignant melanoma with DTIC and BCG. N Eng J Med 1974; 291:592.

9. Kaufman SD, Cosimi AB, Wood WC, Carey RW. Adjuvant therapy in malignant melanoma: A trial of immunotherapy, chemotherapy, and combined treatment, Recent Results Cancer Res 1979; 68:380.

10. Banzet P, Jacquillat C, Civatte J, et al. Adjuvant chemotherapy in the management of primary melanoma. Cancer 1978; 41:1240.

11. Hill II GJ, Moss SE, Golomb FM, et al. DTIC and combination therapy for melanoma: III DTIC surgical adjuvant study COG Protocol 7040. Cancer 1981; 47:2556.

12. Tranum BL, Dixon D, Quagliana J, et al. Lack of benefit of adjunctive chemotherapy in stage I malignant melanoma: A Southwest Oncology Group Study. Cancer Treat Rep 1987; 71:643.

13. Karakousis CP, Emrich LJ. Adjuvant chemotherapy of recurrent malignant melanoma with nitrosourea based protocol. Proc Am Soc Clin Oncol 1989; 8:285.

14. Morton DL, Eilber FR, Malmgren RA. Immunologic factors which influence response to immunotherapy in malignant melanoma. Surgery 1970; 68:158.

15. Cunningham TJ, Schoenfeld D, Nathanson L. et al. A controlled ECOG study of adjuvant therapy with BCG or BCG plus DTIC in patients with stage I and II malignant melanoma. In: immunotherapy of human cancer (W.D. Terry, S.A. Rosenberg eds.). New York: Excerpta Medica, 1982:271.

16. Morton DL, Holmes EC, Eilber FR, et al. Adjuvant immunotherapy of malignant melanoma: Results of a randomized trial in patients with lymph node metastases. In: Immunotherapy of human cancer (W.D. Terry, SA Rosenberg, eds). New York: Excerpta Medica, 1982; 245.

17. O'Connor TPF, Labandter HB, Hiles RW, et al. A clinical trial of BCG immunotherapy as an adjunct to surgery in the treatment of primary malignant melanoma. B Surg 1978; 31:317.

18. Pinsky CM, Hirshaut Y, Wanebo HJ, et al. Randomized trial of bacillus Calmette-Guerin (percutaneous administration) as surgical adjuvant immunotherapy for patients with stage II melanoma. Ann NY Acad Sci 1976; 277:187.

19. Kaiser LR, Burk MW, Morton DL. Adjuvant therapy for malignant melanoma. Surg Clin N Am 1981; 61:1249.

20. Israel L. Report on 414 cases of human tumors treated with corynbacteria. In: *Corynebacterium parvum* applications in experimental and clinical oncology (B.N. Halpern, ed.). New York: Plenum Press, 1975:389.

21. Balch CM, Smalley RV, Bartolucci AA. A randomized prospective clinical trial of adjuvant immunotherapy in 260 patients with clinically localized melanoma (stage I): Prognostic factors analysis and preliminary results of immunotherapy. Cancer 1982; 49:1079.

22. Thatcher N, Mene A, Banerjee SS. Randomized study of *Corynebacterium parvum* adjuvant therapy following surgery for (stage II) malignant melanoma. Br J Surg 1986; 73:111.

23. Lipton A, Harvey HA, Lawrence B, et al. *Corynebacterium parvum* versus BCG adjuvant immunotherapy in human malignant melanoma. Cancer 1983; 51:57.

24. Lipton A, Harvey HA, Balch CM, et al. *Corynebacterium parvum* versus bacille Calmette-Guerin adjuvant immunotherapy of stage II malignant melanoma. J Clin Oncol 1991; 9:1151.

25. Jacquillat C, Banzet P, Civatte J, et al. Adjuvant chemotherapy or chemoimmunotherapy in the management of primary malignant melanoma of level III, IV, or V. Recent Cancer Res 1979; 68:346.

26. Wood WC, Cosimi AB, Carey RW, et al. Randomized trial of

adjuvant therapy for high risk primary malignant melanoma. Surgery 1978; 83:677.

27. Wood WC, Cosimi AB, Carey RW, Kaufman SD. Adjuvant therapy in stage I and II-melanoma. In: Immunotherapy of human cancer (W.D. Terry and S.A. Rosenberg, eds.). New York: Excerpta Medica, 1982:265.

28. Terry WD, Hodes RJ, Rosenberg SA, et al. Treatment of stage I and II malignant melanoma with adjuvant immunotherapy or chemotherapy: Preliminary analysis of a prospective randomized trial. In: Immunotherapy of human cancer (W.D. Terry and S.A. Rosenberg, eds.). New York: Excerpta Medica, 1982:251.

29. Quagliana J, Tranum B, Neidhardt J, et al. Adjuvant chemotherapy with BCNU, Hydrea, and DTIC (BHD) with or without immunotherapy (BCG) in high risk melanoma patients: A SWOG study. Proc Amer Soc Clin Oncol 1980; 21:399.

30. Cunningham TJ, Schoenfeld D, Nathanson L, et al. A controlled ECOG study of adjuvant therapy in patients with stage I & II malignant melanoma. In: Adjuvant therapy of cancer II (E. Jones and S.E. Salmon, eds.). New York: Grune and Stratton, 1979:507.

31. Quirt I, Kersey P, Baker M, et al. A comparison of adjuvant chemoimmunotherapy with observation alone in patients with poor prognosis primary malignant melanoma and completely resected recurrent melanoma. Proc Amer Soc Clin Oncol 1980; 21:472.

32. Quirt IC, DeBoer G, Kersey PA, et al. Randomized controlled trial of adjuvant chemoimmunotherapy with DTIC and BCG after complete excision of primary melanoma with a poor prognosis or melanoma metastases. Can Med Assoc H 1983; 28:929.

33. Veronesi U, Adamus J, Aubert C, et al. A randomized trial of adjuvant chemotherapy and immunotherapy in cutaneous melanoma. N Eng J Med 1982; 307:913.

34. Balch CM, Murray D, Present C, et al. Ineffectiveness of adjuvant chemotherapy using DTIC and cyclophosphamide in patients with resectable metastatic malignant melanoma. Surgery 1984; 95:454.

35. Sterchi JM, Ewells HB, Case LD, et al. A randomized trial of

adjuvant chemotherapy and immunotherapy in stage I and stage II cutaneous melanoma. Cancer 1985; 55:707.

36. Karakousis CP, Emrich LJ. Adjuvant treatment of malignant melanoma with DTIC + Estracyt or BCG. J Surg Oncol 1987; 36:235.

37. Misset JL, Delgado M, De Vassal F, et al. Immunotherapy or chemoimmunotherapy as adjuvant treatment for malignant melanoma: A G.I.F. trial. In: Adjuvant therapy of cancer IV (S.E. Jones and S.E. Salmon, eds.). New York: Grune and Stratton, 1984:557.

38. Czarnetzki BM, Macher E, Behrendt H, Lejeune F. Current status of melanoma chemotherapy and immunotherapy. Recent Results Cancer Res 1982; 80:264.

39. Lejeune FJ, Macher E, Kleeberg U, et al. An assessment of DTIC versus levamisole or placebo in the treatment of high-risk stage I patients after surgical removal of a primary melanoma of skin: A phase III adjuvant study: EORTC protocol 18761. Eur J Cancer Clin Oncol 1988; 24:881.

40. Spitlen LE. A randomized trial of levamisole versus placebo as adjuvant therapy in malignant melanoma. J Clin Oncol 1991; 9:736.

41. Quirt IC, Shelley WE, Pater JL, et al. Improved survival in patients with poor-prognosis malignant melanoma treated with adjuvant levamisole: A phase III study by the National Cancer Institute of Canada Clinical Trial Group. J Clin Oncol 1991; 9:729.

42. Cumberlin R, De Moss E, Lassus M, et al. Isolation perfusion for malignant melanoma of the extremity. J Clin Oncol 1985; 3:1022.

43. Baas PC, Hoekstras HJ, Koops HS, et al. Isolated regional perfusion in the treatment of subungual melanoma. Arch Surg 1989; 124:373.

44. Rege VB, Leone LA, Soderberg CH, et al. Adjuvant perfusion chemotherapy of cutaneous malignant melanoma with minimum 5-year follow-up. In: Adjuvant therapy of cancer V (S.E. Jones and S.E. Salmon, eds.). New York: Grune and Stratton, 1987:671.

45. Franklin HR, Koops HS, Oldhoff J, et al. To perfuse or not to perfuse? A retrospective comparative study to evaluate the

effect of adjuvant isolated regional perfusion in patients with stage I extremity melanoma with a thickness of 1.5 mm or greater. J Clin Oncol 1988; 6:701.

46. Ghussen F, Nagel K, Groth W, et al. A prospective randomized study of regional extremity perfusion in patients with malignant melanoma. Ann Surg 1984; 200:764.

47. Hafstom L, Rudenstam CM, Blomquist E, et al. Regional hyperthermic perfusion with melphalan after surgery for recurrent malignant melanoma of the extremities. J Clin Oncol 1991; 9:2091.

Part IV
Therapy of Advanced Metastatic Melanoma

9

THE ROLE OF CYTOTOXIC CHEMOTHERAPEUTIC AGENTS EITHER ALONE OR IN COMBINATION WITH BIOLOGICAL RESPONSE MODIFIERS

Michael B. Atkins

Beth Israel Deaconess Medical Center and
Harvard Medical School
Boston, Massachusetts

I. INTRODUCTION

Melanoma poses an increasingly important health problem. The incidence of melanoma is increasing at a rate that exceeds all other solid tumors and is approaching 30 per 100,000 in some populations. It is estimated that, by the end of this decade, the lifetime risk of developing a malignant melanoma in the United States will reach 1 in 75 (1). Fortunately, an increasingly large percentage of melanomas are being detected in early stages (stages I and IIA), at which time wide local excision is likely to be curative. In addition, adjuvant therapy with interferon alpha 2B has improved the prognosis for patients with higher-risk lesions (stages IIB and III) (2). While surgery with or without adjuvant interferon can be curative in stage I, II or III disease, a large number of patients with deep primary lesions or nodal involvement are destined to develop distant metastases.

The outlook for patients with melanoma metastases beyond the regional lymph nodes is bleak. Median survival in most series in measured in months. Metastases often involve multiple sites, including skin, lung, liver, bone, bowel, brain, adrenal, kidneys, and heart and can be associated with considerable morbidity (3). Although the benefit of systemic treatment is generally limited, occasional durable complete responses can be achieved. Several treatment options exist, including a variety of cytotoxic chemotherapeutic agents and biological response modifiers; and many promising new approaches are under investigation. This chapter will review the clinical experience with cytotoxic chemotherapy administered either as single agents, in combination chemotherapy regimens, or in combination with biologic response modifiers in patients with metastatic melanoma.

II. SINGLE-AGENT CYTOTOXIC CHEMOTHERAPY FOR METASTATIC MELANOMA

The activity of various chemotherapeutic agents against metastatic melanoma is summarized in Table 1. The agents with greatest antitumor effects include dacarbazine (DTIC®) platinum analogs, nitrosoureas, and tubular toxins.

TABLE 1

Active Single-Agent Chemotherapy for Metastatic Melanoma

Agent (Ref.)	No. of evaluable patients	No. of CR + PR (%)	95% CI (%)
Dacarbazine (DTIC)	1936	382 (20)	18–22
Temozolomide (8)	56	12 (21)	11–32
Carmustine (BCNU)	122	22 (18)	11–25
Lomustine (CCNU)	270	35 (13)	9–17
Fotemustine	153	37 (24)	17–31
Cisplatin	188	43 (23)	17–29
Carboplatin	43	7 (16)	5–27
Vincristine	52	6 (12)	3–20
Vinblastine	62	8 (13)	5–21
Vindesine	273	39 (14)	10–18
Paclitaxel (Taxol)	65	12 (18)	9–28
Docetaxel (Taxotere) (23)	26	4 (15)	2–29
Dibromodulcitol	205	28 (14)	9–18
Detorubicin	42	8 (19)	7–31
Piritrexim	31	7 (23)	8–37

CR = complete response; PR = partial response; 95% CI = confidence interval for response rates.
Source: Ref. 3.

A. Dacarbazine and Temozolomide

Dacarbazine is the most active single agent, with a response rate of approximately 20% (3–5), and it remains the only FDA-approved cytotoxic drug for metastatic melanoma. Patients with involvement limited to skin, subcutaneous tissue, lymph nodes, and, occasionally, lung respond most frequently, and rare (1–2%) durable complete responses can be observed (6). Unfortunately, the vast majority of tumor responses are partial and the median response duration is only 4–6 months (3). Dacarbazine is generally well tolerated with major side effects being limited to nausea and vomiting. Bone-marrow suppression is usually only modest, and alopecia and fatigue are usually minimal, allowing most patients to maintain relatively normal function while receiving therapy. Typical schedules for dacarbazine are 200 mg/m^2 intravenously for 5 days, every 3 to 4 weeks or 850–1000 mg/m^2 intravenously on one day, every 3 to 4 weeks. Response rates and response duration do not appear to be affected by administration schedule. The advent of powerful new antiemetic agents (particularly 5-HT$_3$ antagonists) has significantly reduced the emetogenic effect of dacarbazine, enabling the more convenient one-day, every-three-weeks schedule to be administered in an outpatient setting to most patients.

An analog of dacarbazine, temozolomide, has recently been developed. At physiologic pH, temozolomide chemically degrades to MTIC (methyl triazemoimidazole carboxamide), the active metabolite of dacarbazine, and a process that, in contrast to DTIC, does not require metabolic activation (7). This agent has the potential advantages of being absorbed orally and possessing excellent central nervous system (CNS) penetration. In a Phase II study by the Cancer Research Campaign, temozolomide was well tolerated and produced objective responses in 21% of patients with metastatic melanoma, including 5% complete responses (8).

One of 4 patients with cerebral metastases responded. Temozolomide is currently being compared to dacarbazine in a large European study and, because of its excellent CNS penetration, is being investigated in melanoma patients with newly documented cerebral metastases. In addition, its oral administration route should allow for the examination of novel treatment schedules (such as multiple dose/day or prolonged daily administration) that are not possible with intravenous dacarbazine. Whether temozolomide will prove superior to dacarbazine in any clinical setting remains to be determined.

B. Platinum Analogs

Cisplatin and carboplatin have also shown modest activity in patients with metastatic melanoma. Single-agent cisplatin has been tested at doses of up to 200 mg/m^2, with response rates in the range of 0–53% (mean response rate = 15–20%) (3,9–11). Although no definite dose-response relationship exists for single-agent cisplatin in melanoma, some suggestion of dose dependency is evident from a review of a single-arm studies. Single-agent cisplatin given at doses of up to 150 mg/m^2 in combination with WR-2721, a thiol derivative that is postulated to protect normal host tissues, produced responses in 53% of patients (11). Unfortunately, responses were all partial, and median response duration was only 4 months. A Phase II randomized study of cisplatin 120 mg/m^2 or cisplatin 150 mg/m^2 with WR-2721 conducted by the Eastern Cooperative Oncology Group (ECOG) confirmed that both regimens were active but produced unacceptable renal, gastrointestinal, and ototoxicity (12). Carboplatin has been less extensively tested in metastatic melanoma. Although some responses have been seen in single-agent studies (13), its value relative to cisplatin, dacarbazine, or other single agents remains to be determined.

C. Nitrosoureas

The nitrosoureas carmustine (BCNU), lomustine (CCNU), and semustine (methyl CCNU) have overall response rates of 13–18% (3,4,14–16). Hematologic toxicity and alopecia are more significant with these compounds than with dacarbazine. Although their ability to cross the blood–brain barrier might theoretically offer an advantage for patients with cerebral metastases, a meaningful impact upon CNS disease generally has not been observed. Furthermore, the prolonged thrombocytopenia associated with these agents enhance the risk of hemorrhage into the CNS lesions, with potentially dire consequences. Fotemustine is a chloroethyl nitrosourea which rapidly crosses the blood–brain barrier, possibly through an amino acid transport system. It has been extensively studied in Europe. Initial trials have reported significant activity in patients with metastatic melanoma, including responses in up to 25% of patients with cerebral metastases, but more recent multicenter studies conducted by the EORTC have failed to confirm activity beyond other nitrosoureas (17–20). Although fotemustine is considered first-line therapy in some European countries, it is currently unavailable in the United States. How fotemustine compares with dacarbazine or temozolomide—or how it can be best incorporated into combination therapy regimens (see below)—remains to be determined.

D. Microtubular Toxins

Agents that interfere with microtubular function and cell mitoses, the vinca alkaloids and taxanes, have also shown activity in metastatic melanoma. Vindesine, vinblastine, and vincristine have shown modest activities as single agents (12–14% response rate) (3,21), and the latter two have been used widely in some combination regimens (see below). Paclitaxel and docetaxel have produced responses in about 15% of patients in Phase II trials (22,23). Despite this modest activity, the relative ease of administration of paclitaxel and its unique mechanism of action—inhibition of microtubule disassembly—have prompted its use as second- or third-line therapy and its upfront investigation in combination with platinum analogs. The value of the vinca alkaloids and taxanes, either alone or in combination, in metastatic melanoma remains to be established.

III. COMBINATION CHEMOTHERAPY FOR METASTATIC MELANOMA

A variety of combination chemotherapy regimens have produced response rates of 30–50% in single-institution Phase II trials involving patients with metastatic melanoma (see Table 2). Pivotal Phase III trials comparing various cytotoxic chemotherapy regimens are highlighted in Table 3.

A. Dacarbazine/Nitrosourea Combinations

Two regimens involving dacarbazine and a nitrosourea, BHD (BCNU, hydroxyurea, and dacarbazine), and BOLD (bleomycin, vincristine, CCNU, and dacarbazine), were reported to produce responses in 30–40% of patients (24,25). The contributions of either hydroxyurea or bleomycin to the activity of either of these regimens remains conjectural, as neither has shown significant single-agent activity. The BHD regimen produced a superior response rate relative to dacarbazine and bacille Calmette-Guerin (BCG) (31% vs 18%) in a Southwest Oncology Group (SWOG) trial, but overall survival was not improved (26). Subsequent investigation of the BOLD regimen produced response rates in the 4–20% range (27). Perhaps, consequently, this regimen has never been compared directly to dacarbazine alone.

TABLE 2
Promising Combination Cytotoxic Chemotherapy Regimens
in Metastatic Melanoma

Regimen	Doses	Response rate	Ref.
BHD	BCNU[a] 150 mg/m² Day 1	27%	(24)
	Hydroxyurea 1480 mg/m²/d po D1–5	31%	(26)
	DTIC 150 mg/m²/d D1–5;		
	repeat every 28 days		
BOLD	Bleomycin 15 μ D1, 4		
	Vincristine 1 mg/m²D1, 4	40%	(25)
	CCNU[a] 80 mg/m² D1	4–20%	(27)
	DTIC 200 mg/m² D1–5;		
	repeat every 28 days		
CDDP/DTIC	Cisplatin 50 mg/m²/d D1–3	53%	(28)
	DTIC 350 mg/m²/d D1–3;	20%	(31)
	repeat every 28 days		
CVD	Cisplatin 20 mg/m²/d D1–4	40%	(29)
	Vinblastine 1.5 mg/m²/d D1–4	20%	(32)
	DTIC 800 mg/m² D1;		
	repeat every 3 weeks		
CBDT	Cisplatin 25 mg/m²/d D1–3	55%	(30)
	BCNU[a] 150 mg/m² D1	40%	(33)
	DTIC 220 mg/m²/d D 1–3	51%	(34)
	Tamoxifen 20 mg po q.d.;		
	repeat every 3 weeks		

[a]Given every other cycle.

B. Cisplatin/Dacarbazine Combinations

Three of the most active combination chemotherapy regimens involve cisplatin and dacarbazine. These include the two-drug high-dose combination reported by Murren et al. (28), the three-drug combination of cisplatin/vinblastine/dacarbazine (CVD) developed by Legha et al. (29), and the four-drug combination of cisplatin/BCNU/dacarbazine and

TABLE 3

Randomized Comparisons of Cytotoxic Chemotherapy Regimens
in Metastatic Melanoma

Trial design	Institution (Ref.)	Result/status
BHD vs. dacarbazine + BCG	Southwest Oncology Group (26)	BHD had better RR; overall survival not improved
CVD vs. dacarbazine	M.D. Anderson Cancer Center (32)	RR: CVD 24%, DTIC 11%; p = 0.17 Survival: CVD 27 weeks, DTIC 21 weeks; p = 0.45
CDBT vs. dacarbazine	Eastern Cooperative Oncology Group and MSKCI	Underway

tamoxifen (CBDT) developed by Del Prete et al. and frequently referred to as the "Dartmouth regimen" (30) (see Table 2).

Murren et al. (28) reported a response rate of 53% with acceptable toxicity for the intensive combination of cisplatin 50 mg/m^2/day plus dacarbazine 350 mg/m^2/day for 3 days; however, this regimen displayed much less activity in a subsequent study (31). The CVD regimen produced responses in 40% of 50 patients with 4% CR and median response duration of 9 months (29). In a randomized multi-institutional trial comparing CVD to dacarbazine alone the CVD arm was associated with increases in response rate, response duration, and survival, which at the time of initial publication were not statistically significant (32).

The four-drug CBDT (Dartmouth) regimen produced responses in 46% of 141 patients tested in serial Phase II trials (16 CR and 49 PR) (95% confidence interval, 38–54%) (33). Median response duration was 7 months, and mean survival was about 11 months. Toxicity was generally greater than that observed with dacarbazine alone and included frequent nausea and vomiting, hypomagnesemia, anemia, and, occasionally, severe neutropenia and thrombocytopenia. The hematologic toxicities appeared to be related to cumulative dose, especially for BCNU. In addition, a high incidence of deep venous thrombosis and pulmonary embolism was noted and attributed to the tamoxifen. The inclusion of tamoxifen, however, appeared to be essential, as response rates fell to 10% when the tamoxifen was omitted (34). These encouraging results have prompted many oncologists in the United States to use this regimen as first-line therapy, despite the absence of prospectively randomized trials showing superiority of this regimen to dacarbazine alone. This approach is called into question by two recently completed large group trials. A randomized Phase III NCI–Canada study comparing CBDT to CBD alone showed response rates of only 26% and 21%, respectively (35), and a recently completed phase III trial comparing CBDT to Melacine™ vaccine has shown a response rate of only 13% for the CBDT arm (36). In light of these mixed results, the determination of the true benefit associated with the CBDT relative to dacarbazine alone must await the completion of a randomized Phase III trial currently underway at several institutions and within ECOG.

C. Role of Tamoxifen in Combination Chemotherapy Regimens

Although response rates reported for tamoxifen as a single agent in metastatic malignant melanoma are disappointing (37–40), several investigators have reported its benefit in combination with cytotoxic chemotherapy (33,34). The benefit of tamoxifen in this setting has been attributed to the potentiation of the action of cytotoxic chemotherapy rather than to its purported antiestrogenic effects. Most of these studies involved tamoxifen in combination with multiple other drugs in nonrandomized or, as mentioned previously (34), sequential cohort fashion—making it impossible to accurately assess the true contribution of tamoxifen. In 1992, Cocconi et al. reported the results of a prospective randomized trial of dacarbazine versus dacarbazine + tamoxifen which indicated that the combination therapy was more effective (41). A 28% response rate was reported in patients receiving dacarbazine + tamoxifen, compared to only a 12% response rate in patients treated with dacarbazine alone. Furthermore, median survival was improved from 23 weeks for dacarbazine alone to 41 weeks (31 weeks in men, 71 weeks in women) for combination therapy (p = 0.009). Except for a possibly increased risk of DVT and/or pulmonary embolus in the tamoxifen arm, these benefits were achieved without significant additional toxicity. Unfortunately, several other studies have refuted these results (see Table 4). As mentioned previously, a randomized Phase III trial by the NCI–Canada Clinical Trial Group showed no advantage for the addition of tamoxifen to CBD chemotherapy (35). In addition, other randomized studies showed no advantage for the addition of tamoxifen to either CVD plus interferon (42) or the combination of carboplatin and dacarbazine (43). Finally, a large-scale, four-arm ECOG trial tested the potential benefit of adding tamoxifen to either dacarbazine alone, in a fashion analogous to the Cocconi study, or dacarbazine plus interferon alpha (see below) in patients with metastatic melanoma. This 2 × 2 factorial design trial showed no advantage for the addition of tamoxifen to either regimen in terms of survival (9 months), time to progression (2.3 months), or response rates of the various combinations (44).

In conclusion, although several recent studies using a combination of dacarbazine and a variety of other agents have shown increased response rates, at the present time there is no compelling evidence that any of these combinations is superior to single-agent dacarbazine. The significant

TABLE 4
Tamoxifen in Cytotoxic Chemotherapy Combinations:
Randomized Trials

Design	Institution	Results/conclusion	Source
DTIC +/– Tam	Italian Oncology Group	DTIC + Tam significantly better	Cocconi et al. (41)
CBD +/– Tam	NCI Canada	No difference	Rusthoven et al. (35)
CVD/IFN +/– Tam	M.D. Anderson Cancer Center	No difference	Legha et al. (42)
Carb/DTIC +/– Tam	Pittsburgh Cancer Institute	No difference	Ferri et al. (43)
DTIC +/– Tam or DTIC + IFN +/– Tam	Eastern Cooperative Oncology Group	No difference	Falkson et al. (44)

Tam = tamoxifen; CBD = cisplatin, BCNU, DTIC; CVD = cisplatin, vinblastine, DTIC; Carb = carboplatin

toxicity associated with many of these combination regimens, in comparison to single-agent dacarbazine, further emphasizes the importance of documenting the benefit of these regimens in Phase III trials.

IV. HIGH-DOSE CHEMOTHERAPY AND ABMT IN METASTATIC MELANOMA

The activity of some alkylating agents and the apparent dose–response relationship for cisplatin in metastatic melanoma has prompted several investigators to look at the role of high-dose therapy with autologous bone marrow rescue in this disease. Preparative regimens have included melphalan, BCNU, thiotepa, and carboplatin, or combinations of alkylating agents (3,4,27,36,45–47). Although response rates as high as 80% have been observed, responses have been largely partial and short-lived with very few long-term survivors. In light of the significant toxicity associated with these approaches and the lack of durable benefit, high-dose chemotherapy cannot be recommended as a standard therapy for patients with metastatic melanoma.

V. IMMUNOTHERAPY FOR METASTATIC MELANOMA

A variety of clinical and laboratory observations have suggested that host immunologic mechanisms may occasionally influence the course of melanoma and have fostered interest in the use of biologic response modifier therapy in metastatic disease. During the past decade, two biological agents, interferon (IFN) alpha and Interleukin-2 (IL-2) have shown reproducible single-agent antitumor activity against metastatic melanoma. Both IL-2 and IFN alpha have produced response rates in the 15–20% range (48,49). High-dose IL-2 therapy, administered by IV bolus, either alone or in combination with LAK cells, has produced durable complete responses in approximately 5% of patients (50–52). Although appropriate randomized studies have not been performed, in general the overall response rate, quality, and duration of responses is superior with high-dose IL-2 than with either lower dose IL-2 or IFN alpha. Even within a group of patients all receiving high-dose IL-2, response has been correlated significantly with the amount of IL-2 administered (53). Responses are seen even in patients refractory to cytotoxic chemotherapy, indicating a distinct mechanism of action. Comparable response rates have been reported when IL-2 was administered by continuous infusion (54), although others could not confirm this level of activity (55).

Unfortunately, high-dose IL-2 regimens are associated with significant multiorgan systemic toxicity restricting their use to specialized hospital units capable of providing ICU-level care (56). Although in vitro and preclinical data showed synergy (57) and early clinical trials were promising (58), the combination of IL-2 and IFN alpha, at maximum tolerated doses, has not been proved to be superior to high-dose IL-2 alone (59). Despite extensive investigations, the role, if any, for specific vaccine immunotherapy in metastatic melanoma remains to be established. The value of these more antigen-specific approaches as well as other biologic approaches in the treatent of metastatic and high-risk melanoma are discussed in considerably more detail in the subsequent chapter. The role of these agents in combination with cytotoxic chemo-therapy is discussed below.

VI.   BIOCHEMOTHERAPY REGIMENS FOR METASTATIC MELANOMA

A.   Interferon-Based Biochemotherapy Combinations

Several recent studies have examined the value of adding interferon alpha to cytotoxic chemotherapy. The most promising results were reported by Falkson et al. (60). In a small, randomized trial comparing dacarbazine plus IFN to dacarbazine alone, they observed 12 CR and 4 PR in 30 patients on the combination arm compared with 2 CR and 4 PR in 30 patients treated with dacarbazine alone. Median response durations were 9 months with dacarbazine + IFN alpha and only 2.5 months with dacarbazine alone. Patients receiving dacarbazine + IFN had a median survival rate of 17.6 months versus 9.6 months. The dacarbazine + interferon schedule appeared to be well tolerated, with only 3 patients, having treatment discontinued because of toxicity. Unfortunately, three other randomized trials have not shown an advantage for the addition interferon to dacarbazine (61–63) (see Table 5). These trials

TABLE 5
Randomized Trials of DTIC +/− Interferon alpha in Metastatic Melanoma

Source	Regimens	No. of patients	No. of responses Complete	No. of responses Partial	Response rate (%)
Falkson et al. (60)	DTIC	30	2	4	20
	IFN-α 15 MU/m² IV M-F × 3 week then DTIC + IFN-α 10 MU/m² sc t.i.w.	30	12	4	53[a]
Thompson et al. (61)	DTIC	83	2	12	17
	DTIC (200–800)[b] + IFN-α 9 MU/m²d/SQ	87	6	12	21
Bajetta et al. (62)	DTIC	82	4	12	20
	DTIC + IFN-α 9 MU/d SQ	76	6	15	28
	3 MU t.i.w.	84	6	13	23
Kirkwood et al. (63)	DTIC	24		5[c]	21
	DTIC + IFN 30 MU/m² t.i.w.	21		4[c]	19
Falkson et al. (44)	DTIC +/− Tam	126	3	17	16
	DTIC +/− Tam + IFN[d]	129	7	19	20

DTIC = dacarbazine; IV = intravenous; SQ = subcutaneous; t.i.w. = 3 × per week.
[a]P <.05 v DTIC alone.
[b]The dose of DTIC was 200 mg/m² on the first course, 400 mg/m² on the second course, and 800 mg/m² on the third course.
[c]Responses not subcategorized.
[d]As in Ref. 60.

differ significantly from the Falkson trial, however, in that they did not include a high-dose intravenous interferon induction phase. The recently completed four-arm Phase III randomized ECOG trial (EST 3690) described previously (44) also evaluated the benefit of interferon alpha, administered according to the Falkson schedule, added to either dacarbazine alone or dacarbazine plus tamoxifen. Unfortunately, the addition of interferon alpha was associated with significant toxicity (18% incidence of life-threatening toxicity) and failed to enhance either the response rate, the time to treatment failure, or survival relative to either control arm (44).

In general, results of Phase II trials of IFN alpha added to either other chemotherapy agents (cisplatin, vinca alkaloids, nitrosoureas), CVD, or the Dartmouth regimen have not produced sufficient increments in response rates to warrant Phase III testing (42,64–68). Perhaps the one exception is a study by Pyrhonen et al. evaluating the combination of BOLD plus IFN-α. This regimen produced responses in 62% of 45 patients including 6 (13%) complete remissions (69). Curiously, intermittent dosing of interferon appeared to yield better results than uninterrupted dosing. While this promising result merits further evaluation, the value of interferon alpha in combination biochemotherapy regimens remains to be established.

B. IL-2–Based Biochemotherapy Combinations

A number of investigators have studied combinations of cytotoxic chemotherapy with IL-2–based immunotherapy in metastatic melanoma. IL-2 plus dacarbazine combinations have resulted in considerably more toxicity while yielding response rates of only 13–33%, which clearly are not superior to dacarbazine alone (68–71). More encouraging results have been observed in studies which combine cisplatin-based chemotherapy with either high-dose IL-2 alone or lower doses of IL-2 combined with interferon alpha (72–77). The most intensively studied regimens are listed in Table 6, and results

TABLE 6
Promising Biochemotherapy Regimens

Source	Regimen	Comments
Khayat et al. (76)	CDDP 100 mg/m^2 Day 1 IL-2 18 MIU/m^2 CIV D3–6 and 17–21 IFN 9 MIU/m^2 SC t.i.w +/– Tam 40 mg/m^{2}d –4 to +5 repeat q 3 weeks	85% of patients had prior chemotherapy Tam increased toxicity
Legha and Buzaid (75) Sequential[a] CVD Bio	CDDP 20 mg/m^2/d D2–5 Vinblastine 1.6 mg/m^2/d D1–5 DTIC 800 mg/m^{2}D1 IL-2 9 MIU/m^2/d × 96 hours IFN 5 mg/m^2/d × 5d; repeat q 28 days	CVD first better than Bio first (66% vs. 40%)
Richards et al. (74)	CDDP 25 mg/m^2/d D1–3 DTIC 220 mg/m^2/d D1–3 BCNU[b] 150 mg/m^2 D1 Tam 20 mg/m^2 qd IL-2 4.5 MIU/m^{2}IV and IFN 6.0 MI/m^2 sc D4–8 and 17–21; repeat q 28 days	High incidence of vitiligo in responders
Atkins et al. (78)	CDDP 50 mg/m^2/d D1–3 DTIC 350 mg/m^2/d D1–3 IL-2 600,000 IU/kg IV q8h D12–16 and 26–30	Significant toxicity multicenter trial
Flaherty et al. (79)	CDDP 100 mg/m^2 D1 DTIC 750 mg/m^2 D1 IL-2 MIU/m^2/d D12–16 and 19–23	

[a]Compared CVD + Bio Days 6–10 and 17–21 vs. Bio + CVD.
[b]Every other cycle.

are displayed and summarized in Table 7. Composite results in nearly 400 patients show a response rate of approximately 50%, with 10–20% complete responses, a median response duration of 6–8 months, and a median survival of 11–12 months. Ten percent of all patients appeared to have achieved durable complete responses. In contrast to either chemotherapy or immunotherapy alone, responses were seen at all disease sites with equal frequency, and no clear dose-response relationship for either IL-2 or cisplatin was apparent. Interesting observations from individual studies included: responses in patients with prior chemotherapy and the probable requirement for cisplatin to achieve synergy (76); no interference of chemotherapy with ongoing responses produced by IL-2 (77); an apparent advantage if chemotherapy is administered prior to biotherapy (75); and responses seen in patients with CNS metastases and, more frequently, in patients who develop vitiligo (74,76). As is often the case with metastatic melanoma (34,80) isolated CNS relapses occurred in many responding patients (77,78). Nonetheless, the apparent higher response rate and the 10% durable unmaintained CR rate raise the possibility that

TABLE 7
IL-2/Cisplatin–Based Biochemotherapy:
Summary of Metastatic Melanoma Results

Source	N	CR/PR (%)	Duration (months)	Survival (months)
Richards et al. (74)	74	11/30 (55)	8+	11+
Legha and Buzaid (75)	115	25/44 (60)	NA	12
Khayat et al. (76)	111	10/41 (49)	6–14	11
Atkins et al. (77,78)	65	6/20 (40)	5–6	11
Flaherty et al. (79)	32	5/8 (41)	8	10+
Total	397	57/143 (50.3%)[a]		

[a]95% confidence intervals 47–53%

these combination regimens may be superior to either chemotherapy or immunotherapy alone (81). Unfortunately, all these regimens involved extensive in-patient treatment and substantial toxicity, expense and patient time commitment, making more widespread Phase III investigation impractical.

C. Potential Mechanism for Synergistic Interaction for Biochemotherapy

The initial rationale for combining biologic response modifiers and cytotoxic chemotherapy agents was the hope of producing additive antitumor effects. This belief was bolstered by preclinical and anecdotal clinical evidence of non-cross–resistance (82,83). Consequently, efforts were made to administer maximum tolerated dose of component regimens in an alternating fashion. These studies resulted in significant toxicity necessitating long delays between treatment components. Additive responses were observed, and, encouragingly, the cytotoxic chemotherapy did not appear to interfere with ongoing responses induced by IL-2–based immunotherapy (77). This led to efforts to administer the chemotherapy first and to approximate the two treatment components more closely. The higher response rates including responses in typically refractory sites and even in patients who had previously received cytotoxic chemotherapy [76] with this approach, and the lack of a clear dose–response relationship, raised the possibility that synergistic interactions between the cytotoxic and biologic components may be involved.

Proposed mechanisms for such synergy have included cisplatin-mediated augmentation of immune activation or enhancement of tumor antigen presentation (84,85). Alternatively, the biotherapeutic agents could conceivably enhance the cytotoxic effects of cisplatin through release of toxic substances (hydrogen peroxide, IL-1, TNF, etc.) by activated tumor-infiltrating monocytes and/or lymphocytes. This hypothesis is supported by experiments by Braunschweiger et al. with cisplatin and IL-1 alpha (86,87) but requires validation in the setting of IL-2/cisplatin–based biochemotherapy. If a benefit for biochemotherapy relative to chemotherapy alone can be established clinically, then understanding the mechanisms of potential interactions may prove critical to the design of more effective regimens against melanoma and might even allow the application of these concepts to other tumor types.

D. Randomized Trials Involving IL-2/Cisplatin–Based Biochemotherapy

A few large single institutions within the United States and the Melanoma Group within EORTC have initiated Phase III investigations of biochemotherapy regimens. M.D. Anderson has begun a study comparing their sequential CVD/IL2/IFN regimen to CVD alone; and the NCI Surgery Branch has initiated a similar study comparing the combination cisplatin, dacarbazine and tamoxifen, plus high-dose IL-2, and IFN alpha to cisplatin, dacarbazine, and tamoxifen alone (36) (see Table 8). Both of these studies aim to address the direct contribution of IL-2 and interferon alpha to combination cytotoxic chemotherapy. As neither of these regimens are suitable for a cooperative group or community hospital setting, these trials are likely to take a long time to complete, and their results, although scientifically interesting, may be of little practical importance.

In contrast, the EORTC Melanoma Group has examined the value of adding cisplatin to IL-2/IFN biotherapy in a randomized Phase III trial (88). IL-2 was administered using a decrescendo regimen (1 mg/m^2 over 6 hours, followed by 1 mg/m^2 over 12 hours, 1 mg/m^2 over 24 hours, and a

TABLE 8

Phase III Randomized Trials of Biochemotherapy Regimens
in Metastatic Melanoma

Source	Trial design	Status
Legha et al.; M.D. Anderson Cancer Center	Sequential CVD/IL-2/ IFN vs. CVD	Underway
Rosenberg et al.; NCI Surgery Branch	Cisplatin/DTIC/Tam +/− high-dose IL-2/ IFN	Underway
Keilholz et al.; EORTC	Decrescendo IL-2/IFN +/− CDDP	Combination significantly improved response rate; survival data pending
Keilholz et al.; EORTC	DTIC/CDDP/IFN +/− IL-2	Underway
Atkins et al.; Intergroup	Concurrent CVD-IL-2 /IFN vs. CVD	Proposed

maintenance dose of 0.25 mg/m^2 over 24 hours for 3 days) to patients on both treatment arms, while one group of patients also received cisplatin 100 mg/m^2 on day 1. Cycles were repeated at 28-day intervals. Patients were stratified according to pretreatment serum LDH levels and tumor burden. Results showed a significantly higher response rate (36% vs. 15%) in the cisplatin containing arm, irrespective of tumor burden. Median response durations were 6 months in each arm and no difference in impact upon survival could be demonstrated. The EORTC Melanoma Committee has recently initiated a follow-up study in which patients will be randomized to receive cisplatin/DTIC/IFN +/– decrescendo IL-2.

E. Concurrent Biochemotherapy Regimen

In an effort to enhance the practicality of biochemotherapy, Legha et al. developed a regimen in which CVD chemotherapy was administered concurrently with IL-2 and IFN alpha immunotherapy (89). Patients received DTIC 800 mg/m^2 on day 1, cisplatin 20 mg/m^2 on days 1–4, and vinblastine 1.6 mg/m^2 on days 1–5, together with a 96-hour continuous infusion of IL-2 (9 MU/m^2/day) and intermittent IFN alpha. Therapy was administered every 3 weeks in an in-patient setting over 5 days. This regimen produced responses in 33 (11 CR/22 PR) of 53 patients (RR 63%), with a median response duration of 6 months. Recurrence in the central nervous system was the major factor responsible for this short duration of response (36,89,90). Five patients (9%) remain in CR at 24–36 months follow-up.

Although toxicity was reduced in comparison to other biochemotherapy regimens, significant toxicity was still observed. Frequent problems included hypotension requiring pressors and catheter related bacteremia. These problems were more frequent in later cycles of therapy (Legha, et al., personal communication). The use of prolonged indwelling central venous catheters as well as total vinblastine doses > 6 mg/m^2 were felt to be the major contributing factors to the high incidence of bacteremia. It is possible that these side effects could be reduced through minor alterations in the dose modification criteria and supportive measures (i.e., removal of central catheters following each cycle, routine use of prophylactic antibiotics, 20% reduction in vinblastine dose, and early institution of hematopoietic growth factors). These modifications are currently being examined in a pilot study and, if successful in significantly reducing these various toxicities, this regimen may prove suitable for testing within a cooperative group setting in comparison to chemotherapy alone, in a Phase III randomized trial.

F. Outpatient Biochemotherapy Regimens

The observation that the activity of cisplatin and IL-2 based biochemotherapy regimens may be related more to the temporal proximity of the biologic and cytotoxic components than to the actual doses of the individual agents has raised the possibility of developing regimens suitable for outpatient administration. With this in mind, Thompson et al. performed a Phase II trial of outpatient chemoimmunotherapy in patients with metastatic melanoma (91). Patients received BCNU 150 mg/m^2, DTIC 660 mg/m^2, and cisplatin 75 mg/m^2 on day 1, together with tamoxifen 20 mg daily (after a brief loading dose) and IL-2 3 MIU/m^2 subcutaneously on days 3–9, and IFN alpha 2A 3–9 MU subcutaneously days on 3, 5, 7, and 9. Thirty-two patients received 96 cycles of therapy. Nausea and vomiting were the major side effects. Supplemental intravenous hydration was required in 31 cycles, but less the 10% of patients required in-patient hospitalization. Other toxicities were mild and quickly reversible. An overall response rate of 44% (4CR/10 PR) was observed, but follow-up is too short to merit comment on response durability. A similar regimen, omitting the BCNU and tamoxifen and using slightly higher doses of IL-2 either subcutaneously or intravenously, was initiated in the Cytokine Working Group, but was associated with toxicity requiring frequent hospitalizations for intractable nausea, vomiting, and dehydration (Atkins, et al, unpublished observations). Whether these regimens are truly suitable for routine out-patient use, and how they compare to either chemotherapy alone or more thoroughly tested in-patient biochemotherapy regimens, remains to be determined.

VII. CONCLUSIONS

Many different agents appear to have modest antitumor activity against metastatic melanoma; however, despite the promising results of a variety of combination regimens, none have been shown to be superior to dacarbazine alone in large-scale randomized Phase III trials. Biochemotherapy combinations have produced 50% response rates and 10% unmaintained CR rates, suggesting a potential advantage over dacarbazine alone (88). Although these promising results come mostly from single-institution Phase II trials involving highly selected patients, they appear to be remarkably consistent. Phase III trials are clearly necessary to establish the current optimal cytotoxic chemotherapy regimen (CBDT versus dacarbazine) and to determine if there is meaningful benefit achieved from addition of IL-2–based biologic therapy. Recently, several such studies have been initiated or are in the planning stages. It is hoped that these studies will establish a new standard of care for this difficult disease. Nonetheless, even with the best available regimens, the vast majority of patients still succumb to their disease, leaving ample room for improvement. New cytotoxic chemotherapy agents such as temozolomide, fotemustine, and the taxanes offer the promise of reducing the risk of CNS relapse or palliating resistent disease, yet their benefit is likely to be marginal at best. Major advances in the treatment of melanoma will likely require the development of novel biological or immunological approaches such as those described elsewhere in this volume.

REFERENCES

1. Wingo P, Tong T, Bolden S. Cancer statistics, 1995. CA Cancer J Clin 1995; 45:8–30.
2. Kirkwood JM, Strawderman H, Ernstoff MS, Smith TJ, Borden EC, Blum RH. Interferon alfa-2b adjuvant therapy of

high-risk resected cutaneous melanoma: The Eastern Cooperative Oncology Group trial EST 1684. J Clin Oncol 1996; 14: 7–17.

3. Balch CM, Houghton A, Peters LJ. Cutaneous melanoma. In: Devita H, Hellman, Rosenberg Z, eds. Cancer Principles & Practices of Oncology. 4th ed. New York: J.B. Lippincott, 1993:1612.

4. Houghton AN, Legha S, Bajorin DF. Chemotherapy for metastatic melanoma. In: Balch CM, Houghton A, Milton, Sober, Soong, ed. Cutaneous Melanoma. 2nd ed. New York: J.B. Lippincott Company, 1992:498–508.

5. Comis RL. DTIC (NSC-45388) in malignant melanoma: A perspective. Cancer Treat Rep 1976; 64:1123.

6. Hill GJ, Krementz ET, Hill HZ. Dimethyl triazenoimidazole carboxamide and combination therapy for melanoma: Late results after complete response to chemotherapy. Cancer 1984; 53:1299.

7. Stevens MFG, Hickman JA, Langdon SP, et al. Antitumor activity and pharmacokinetics in mice of 8-carbamoyl-3-methylimidazo [5,1-d] 1, 2, 3, 5-tetrazin-4 (3H) one (CCRG) 81045: M&B 39831 A novel drug with potential as an alternative to dacarbazine. Cancer Res 1987; 47:5846–5852.

8. Bleehen NM, Newlands SM, Thatcher LN, Selby P, Calver AH, Rustin GJ, Brampton M, Stevens MFG. Cancer Research Campaign Phase II trial of temozolomide in metastatic melanoma. J Clin Oncol 1995; 13:910–913.

9. Al-Sarraf M, Fletcher W, Oishi N, et al. Cisplatin hydration with and without mannitol diuresis in refractory disseminated malignant melanoma: A Southwest Oncology Group study. Cancer Treat Rep 1982; 66:31.

10. Song SY, Chary KK, Higby DJ, Henderson ES, Klein E. Cisdiamminedichloride platinum (II) in the treatment of metastatic melanoma. Clin Res 1977; 25:411.

11. Glover D, Glick JH, Weiler C, et al. WR2721 and High-Dose Cis-platin: An active combination in the treatment of metastatic melanoma. J Clin Oncol 1987; 5:574.

12. Glover D, Glick JH, et al. Unpublished data.

13. Evans LM, Casper ES, Rosenbluth R. Participating community clinical oncology program investigators: Phase II trial of

carboplastin in advanced malignant melanoma. Cancer Treatment Reports 1987; 71:171.

14. Ramirez G, Wilson W, Grage T, et al. Phase II evaluation of 1,3-bis (2-chloroethyl-nitrosourea) (BCNU: NSC-409962) in patients with solid tumors. Cancer Chemother Rep 1972; 56: 787.

15. Wasserman TH, Slavik M, Carter SK. Review of CCNU in clinical cancer therapy. Cancer Treat Rev 1974; 1:131.

16. Young RC, Canellos GP, Chabner BA, et al. Treatment of malignant melanoma with methyl-CCNU. Cancer Pharmacol Ther 1974; 15:617.

17. Jacquillat C, Khayat D, Banzet P, et al. Final report of the French multicenter Phase II study of the nitrosourea Fotemustine in 153 evaluable patients with disseminated malignant melanoma including patients with cerebral metastases. Cancer 1990; 56:1873.

18. Calabresi F, Aspro M, Becquart D, et al. Multicenter Phase II trial of the single agent Fotemustine in patients with advanced malignant melanoma. Ann Oncol 1991; 2:378.

19. Schallecuter KU, Wenzel E, Bressow FW, et al. Positive phase II study in the treatment of advanced malignant melanoma with fotemustine. Cancer Chemother Pharmacol 1991; 29:85.

20. Khayat D, Avril M, Auclerc G, et al. Clinical value of the nitrosourea fotemustine in disseminated malignant melanoma: Overview on 1022 patients including 144 patients with cerebral metastases. Proc Am Soc Clin Oncol 1993; 12:393.

21. Quagilana JM, Stephens M, Baker LH, Constanzi JJ. Vindesine in patients with metastatic malignant melanoma. A Southwest Oncology Group study. J Clin Oncol 1984; 4:316.

22. Einzig AJ, Hochster H, Wiernik PH, et al. A phase II study of taxol in patients with malignant melanoma. Invest New Drug 1991; 9:59.

23. Bedikian A, Legha S, Jenkins J, Eton O, Buzaid A, Plager C, Papadopoulos N, Benjamin R. Phase II trial of docetaxel in patients with advanced melanoma previously untreated with chemotherapy. Proc ASCO 1995; 14:412.

24. Costanzi JJ, Vaitkevicicus VK, Quagliana JM, Hoogstraten B, Coltman CA Jr., Delaney FC. Combination chemotherapy for disseminated malignant melanoma. Cancer 1975; 35:342.

25. Seigler HF, Lucas VS Jr., Pickett NJ, Huang AT. DTIC, CCNU, bleomycin and vincristine (BOLD) in metastatic melanoma. Cancer 1980; 46:2346.

26. Costanzi JJ, Al-Sarraf M, Groppe C, Bottomley R, Fabian C, Neidhart J. et al. Combination chemotherapy plus BCG in the treatment of disseminated malignant melanoma: A Southwest Oncology Group study. Med Pediatr Oncol 1982; 10:251.

27. Kirkwood J, Agarwala S. Systemic cytotoxic and biological therapy of melanoma. PPO Updates 1993; 7:1–16.

28. Murren JR, DeRosa W, Durivage HJ, et al. High-dose cisplatin plus dacarbazine in the treatment of metastatic melanoma. Cancer 1991; 67:1514–1517.

29. Legha SS, Ring S, Papadopoulos N, Plager C, Chawla S, Benjamin R. A prospective evaluation of a triple-drug regimen containing cisplatin, vinblastine and DTIC (CVD) for metastatic melanoma. Cancer 1989; 64:2024.

30. Del Prete SA, Maurer LH, O'Donnell J, et al. Combination chemotherapy with cisplatin, carmustine, dacarbazine and tamoxifen in metastatic melanoma. Cancer Treat Rep 1984; 68:1403–1405.

31. Steffens TA, Bajorin DF, Lovett DR, et al. A Phase II study of cisplatin (CDDP) and dacarbazine (DTIC) in patients with metastatic melanoma (abstr.) Proc Am Soc Clin Oncol 1991; 10:296.

32. Buzaid AC, Legha S, Winn R, Belt R, Pollock T, Wiseman C, Ensign LG. Cisplatin (C), vinblastine (V), and dacarbazine (D) (CVD) versus dacarbazine alone in metastatic melanoma: Preliminary results of a Phase III Cancer Community Oncology Program (CCOP) trial, Proc ASCO 1993; 12:389.

33. Mastrangelo MJ, Berd D, Bellet RE. Aggressive chemotherapy for melanoma. PPO Updates 1991; 5:1.

34. McClay EF, Mastrangelo MJ, Berd D, Bellet, RE. Effective combination chemo/hormonal therapy for malignant melanoma: Experience with three clinical trials. Int J Cancer 1992; 50:553.

35. Rusthoven J, Quirt I, Iscoe N, McCulloch P, James K, Lochmann R, Jensen J, Burdette-Radoux S, Bodurtha A, Silver H, Verma S, Amitage GR, Zee B, Bennett K. National Can-

cer Institute of Canada Clinical Trials Group, J Clin Oncol 1996; 14:2083–2090.

36. Mitchell MS, Von Eschan KB. Phase III trial of Melacine® melanoma theracine versus combination chemotherapy in the treatment of stage IV melanoma. Proc Asco 1997; 16:494a.

37. Wagstaff J, Thatcher N, Rankin E. et al. Tamoxifen in the treatment of metastatic melanoma. Cancer Treat Rep 1982; 66:1171.

38. Leichman CG, Samson MK, Baker LH. Phase II trial of tamoxifen in malignant melanoma. Cancer Treat Rep 1982; 66:1447.

39. Telhaug R, Klepp O, Bremer O. Phase II study of tamoxifen in patients with metastatic malignant melanoma. Cancer Treat Rep 1982; 66:1437.

40. Creagan ET, Ingle JN, Ahmann DL, et al. Phase II study of high-dose tamoxifen (NSC 180973) in patients with disseminated melanoma. Cancer Treat Rep 1984; 68:1403.

41. Cocconi G, Bella M, Calabresi F, et al. Treatment of metastatic malignant melanoma with dacarbazine plus tamoxifen. N Engl J Med 1992; 327:516–523.

42. Legha S, Ring S, Bedikian A, Eton O, Plager C, Papadopoulos N, Ensign LG, Benjamin RS. Lack of benefit from tamoxifen (T) added to a regimen of cisplatin (C), vinblastine (V), DTIC (D) and alpha interferon (IFN) in patients with metastatic melanoma. Proc ASCO 1993; 12:388.

43. Ferri W, Agarwala SS, Kirkwood JM, Gooding W, Vlock D, Miketic L, Donnell S. carboplatin (C) and dacarbazine (D) ± tamoxifen (T) for metastatic melanoma. Proc ASCO 1994; 13:394.

44. Falkson CI, Ibrahim J, Kirkwood J, Blum R. A randomized phase III trial of dacarbazine (DTIC) versus DTIC + interferon Alfa-2b (IFN) versus DTIC + tamoxifen (TMX) versus DTIC + IFN + TMX in metastatic malignant melanoma: An ECOG trial. Proc ASCO 1996; 15:435.

45. Lazarus HM, Herzig RH, Wolff SN, et al. Treatment of metastatic malignant melanoma with intensive melphalan and autologous bone marrow transplantation. Cancer Treat Rep 1985; 69:473.

46. Wolff SN, Herzig RH, Fay JW, et al. High dose thiotepa with autologous bone marrow transplantation for metastatic melanoma: Results of phase I–II studies of the North Ameri-

can Bone Marrow Transplantation Group. J Clin Oncol 1989; 7:245.

47. Antman K, Eder JP, Elias A, et al. High dose combination alkylating agent preparative regimen with autologous bone marrow support: The Dana-Farber Cancer Institute/Beth Israel Hospital experience. Cancer Treat Rep 1987; 71:119 45.

48. Kirkwood JM. Studies of interferon in the therapy of melanoma. Semin Oncol (suppl 7) 1991; 18:83–89.

49. Sparano JA, Dutcher JP. Interleukin-2 for the treatment of advanced melanoma. Hem/Onc Annals 1993; 1:279–285.

50. Dutcher JP, Creekmore S, Weiss GR, et al. Phase II study of high-dose interleukin-2 and lymphokine activated killer cells in patients with metastatic malignant melanoma. J Clin Oncol 1989; 7:477–485.

51. Parkinson DR, Abrams JS, Wiernik PH, et al. Interleukin-2 Therapy in patients with metastatic malignant melanoma: A Phase II study. J Clin Oncol 1990; 8:1650–1656.

52. Rosenberg SA, Yang JC, Topalian SL, et al. Treatment of 283 consecutive patients with metastatic melanoma or renal cell cancer using high-dose bolus interleukin-2. JAMA 271 (12) 1994; 907–913.

53. Royal RE, Steinberg SM, White De, et al. Correlates of response to IL-2 therapy in patients treated for metastatic renal cancer and melanoma. Cancer J Sci Am 1996; 6:91–98.

54. West WH, Tauer KW, Yanelli JR. et al. Constant-infusion recombinant interleukin-2 and adoptive immunotherapy of advanced cancer. N Engl J of Med 1987; 316:898–905.

55. Dutcher JP, Gaynor ER, Boldt DH, et al. A phase II study of high-dose continuous infusion interleukin-2 with lymphokine activated killer cells. J Clin Oncol 1991; 9:641–648.

56. Margolin K. The clinical toxicities of high-dose interleukin-2. In: Atkins MB, Mier JW, eds. Therapeutic applications of interleukin-2. New York: Marcel Dekker, 1993; 331–362.

57. Cameron RB, McIntosch JK, Rosenberg SA. Synergistic antitumor effects of combination immunotherapy with recombinant interleukin-2 and recombinant hybrid alpha-interferon in the treatment of established murine hepatic metastases. Cancer Res 1988; 48:5810–5817.

58. Rosenberg SA, Lotze MT, Yang JC, et al. Combination therapy

with interleukin-2 and alpha-interferon for the treatment of patients with advanced cancer. J Clin Oncol 1989; 7: 1863–1874.

59. Sparano JA, Fisher RI, Sunderland, et al. Randomized phase III trial of treatment with high-dose interleukin-2 either alone or in combination with interferon alfa-2a in patients with advanced melanoma. J Clin Oncol 1993; 11:1969–1977.

60. Falkson CI, Falkson G, Falkson HC. Improved results with the addition of interferon alpha-2b to dacarbazine in the treatment of patients with metastatic malignant melanoma. J Clin Oncol 1991; 9:1403–1408.

61. Thompson D, Adena M, McLeod GRC, et al. Interferon alfa-2a does not improve response or survival when combined with dacarbazine in metastatic malignant melanoma: Results of a multi-institutional Australian randomized trial QMP8704. Melanoma Res 1993; 3:133–138.

62. Bajetta E, Di Leo A, Zampino M, et al. Multicenter randomized trial of dacarbazine alone or in combination with two different doses and schedules of interferon alfa-2A in the treatment of advanced melanoma. J Clin Oncol 1994; 12:806–811.

63. Kirkwood JM, Ernstoff MS, Giuliano A, et al. Interferon α-2a and dacarbazine in melanoma. J Natl Cancer Inst 1990; 82:1062–1063.

64. Margolin K, Doroshow J, Akman S, et al. Treatment of advanced melanoma with cisdiamminedichloroplatinum (CDDP) and alpha interferon (aIFN). Proc Am Soc Clin Oncol 1990; 9:277.

65. Morton R, Cregan E, Schaid D, et al. Phase III trial of recombinant leukocyte a interferon (IFN-alpha-2a) plus 1,3-bis(2-chloroethyl)-1-nitrosourea (BCNU) and the combination cimetidine with BCNU in patients with disseminated malignant melanoma. Am J Clin Oncol (CCT) 1991; 14:152–155.

66. Smith K, Green J, Eccles J. Interferon alpha-2a and vindesine in the treatment of advanced malignant melanoma. Eur J Cancer 1992; 28:438–441.

67. Stark J, Schulof R, Wiemann M, et al. Alpha interferon and chemo-hormonal therapy in advanced melanoma: A phase I/II NBSG/MAOP study. Proc Am Soc Clin Oncol 1993; 12:392.

68. Schultz M, Buzaid A, Poo W: A Phase II study of interferon-alpha 2b with dacarbazine, cisplatin, camustine, and tamoxifen in metastatic melanoma. Melanoma Res 1995, in press.

69. Pyrhonen S, Hahka-Kemppinen, Muhonen T. A promising interferon plus four-drug regimen for metastatic melanoma. J Clin Oncol 1992; 10:1919–1926.

70. Dillman R, Oldham R, Barth N, et al. Recombinant interleukin-2 and adoptive immunotherapy alternated with dacarbazine therapy in melanoma: A National Biotherapy Study Group trial. J Natl Cancer Inst 1990; 82:1345–1349.

71. Fiedler W, Jasmin C, De Mulder P, et al. A Phase II study of sequential recombinant interleukin-2 followed by dacarbazine in metastatic melanoma. Eur J Cancer 1992; 28:443–446.

72. Flaherty L, Liu P, Fletcher W, et al. Dacarbazine and outpatient interleukin-2 in treatment of metastatic malignant melanoma: A phase II Southwest Oncology Group trial. J Natl cancer Inst 1992; 83:893–894.

73. Stoter G, Aamda S, Rodenhuis S, et al. Sequential administration of recombinant human interleukin-2 and dacarbazine in metastatic melanoma: A multicenter phase II study. J Clin Oncol 1991; 9:1687–1691.

74. Richards JM, Mehta N, Schroeder L, et al. Sequential chemotherapy/immunotherapy for metastatic melanoma. (abstr.) Proc ASCO 1992; 11:346.

75. Legha SS, Buzaid AC. Role of recombinant interleukin-2 in combination with interferon-alfa and chemotherapy in the treatment of advanced melanoma. Semin Oncol (suppl 9) 1993; 20:27–32.

76. Khayat D, Borel C, Tourani JM, et al. Sequential chemoimmunotherapy with cisplatin, interleukin-2 and interferon alfa-2a for metastatic melanoma. J Clin Oncol 1993; 12:2173–2180.

77. Demchak PA, Mier JW, Robert NJ, et al. Interleukin-2 and

high-dose cisplatin in patients with metastatic melanoma: A pilot study. J Clin Oncol 1991; 9:1821–1830.

78. Atkins MB, O'Boyle KR, Sosman JA, et al. Multi-institutional phase II trial of intensive combination chemoimmunotherapy for metastatic melanoma. J Clin Oncol 1994; 12:1553–1560.

79. Flaherty LE, Robinson W, Redman BG, Gonzales R, Martino S, Kraut M, Valdivieso M, and Rudloph AR. A phase II study of dacarbazine and cisplatin in combination with outpatient administered interleukin-2 in metastatic malignant melanoma, Cancer 1993; 71:3520–3525.

80. Mitchell MS. Relapse in the central nervous system in melanoma patients successfully treated by biomodulators. J Clin Oncol 1989; 7:1701–1709.

81. Legha S, Ring S, Eton C, Plager A, Buzaid A, Papadopolous N. Durable complete responses (CR's) in metastatic melanoma treated with biochemotherapy using cisplatin + vinblastine + DTIC (CVD) and IL-2 + interferon-alpha (IFN-α) (abstr). Proc ASCO 1995; 14:412.

82. Sznol M, Longo DL. Chemotherapy drug interactions with biological agents. Semin Oncol 1991; 20:80–93.

83. Richards JM, Gilewski TA, Ramming K, et al. Effective chemotherapy for melanoma after treatment with interleukin-2. Cancer 1992; 69:427–429.

84. Basu S, Sodhi A, Singh S, et al. Up-regulation of induction of lymphokine (IL-2) activated killer (LAK) cell activity by FK-565 and cisplatin. Immunol Lett 1991; 27:199–204.

85. Mizutani Y, Nio Y, Yoshida O. Modulation by cisdiamminedichloroplatinum (II) of the susceptibilities of human T24 lined and freshly separated autologous urinary bladder transitional carcinoma cells to peripheral blood lymphocytes and lymphokine activated killer cells. J Urol 1992; 147:505–510.

86. Braunschweiger P, Bastur V, Santos O, et al. Synergistic anti-tumor activity of cisplatin and interleukin-1 in sensitive and resistant solid tumors. Cancer Res 1993; 53:1091–1097.

87. Braunschweiger P, Bastur V, Santos O. Interleukin-1α induced oxidants increase cisplatin cytotoxicity in squamos

cell carcinoma cells in vitro (abstr.). Proc AACR 1993; 34:466.

88. Keilholz U, Goey SH, Punt CJA, Proebstle T, Salzman R, Schadenforf D, Lienard D, Scheibenbogen C, Eggermont AMM. A randomized trial of IFNα/IL-2 with or without CDDP in advanced melanoma: An EORTC melanoma Cooperative Group trial. Proc ASCO 1996; 15:436.

89. Buzaid AC, Legha SS. Combination of chemotherapy with interleukin-2 and interferon-alfa for the treatment of advanced melanoma. Semin. Oncol 1994; 21:23–28.

90. Legha S, Buzaid AC, Ring S, Bedikian A, Plager C, Eton O, Papadopoulos, Benjamin RS. Improved results of treatment of metastatic melanoma with combined use of biotherapy and chemotherapy (biochemo). Proc ASCO 1994; 13:394.

91. Thompson J, Gold P, Fefer A. Outpatient chemo-immunotherapy for patients with metastatic melanoma. Proc ASCO 1996; 15:433.

10

RADIOSURGERY IN THE MANAGEMENT OF MELANOMA BRAIN METASTASIS

John C. Flickinger, Salvador Somaza,
and Douglas Kondziolka

University of Pittsburgh
Pittsburgh, Pennsylvania

I. INTRODUCTION

Metastasis to the central nervous system has been the cause of death in approximately one third of patients with malignant melanoma (6). If current and future improvements in systemic chemotherapy and immunotherapy lengthen the survival of melanoma patients with systemic disease, untreated microscopic brain metastases likely will become symptomatic in more of these patients. Brain metastases pose a particularly difficult problem in patients being considered for immunotherapy because of the risk of exacerbating intracranial (peritumoral) edema.

Treatment options for melanoma patients with newly diagnosed brain metastases include: supportive medical therapy with corticosteroids and/or anticonvulsants; fractionated low- or high dose whole-brain radiotherapy; surgical resection with or without radiotherapy; and stereotactic radiosurgery with or without fractionated whole-brain radiotherapy.

II. WHOLE-BRAIN RADIOTHERAPY

The prognosis for melanoma patients with solitary or multiple brain metastases undergoing standard whole-brain radiotherapy is poor (3 months in a number of series) (22). Several strategies have been explored to try to improve results after whole-brain radiotherapy for brain metastasis in general and melanoma in particular.

One of the first Radiation Therapy Oncology Group (RTOG) studies investigated different radiation fractionation schedules for whole brain irradiation in 1830 brain metastasis patients (4,10). No differences in median survival were detected among the five different treatment schedules: 20 Gy in five fractions; 30 Gy in 10 or 15 fractions; and 40 Gy in 15 or 20 fractions. Even though 20 Gy in five fractions appeared equally effective, most radiotherapists in the United States treat brain-metastasis patients with whole-brain irradiation to 30 Gy in 10 or 12 fractions because of a concern that larger 4-Gy dose-fractions will lead to an increased risk of delayed neurological deficits. In the RTOG study, ambulatory patients with no systemic metastases had the greatest median survival (28 weeks) compared to nonambulatory patients (11 weeks).

Because malignant melanoma has been observed to be a relatively radioresistant neoplasm that may respond better to large dose-fractions, Vlock et al. compared conventional whole-brain radiotherapy with 30 Gy in 10 fractions (3 Gy per fraction for melanoma brain metastasis) to high-dose per fraction whole-brain radiotherapy (30 Gy in 5 fractions; 6 Gy per fraction) (27). No difference in survival was identified, and progression of brain disease was noted in the majority of patients in this study.

The extent to which brain metastases eventually regrow after conventional radiotherapy has not always been appreciated, since many patients succumb to progression of extracranial metastases and many radiotherapists do not maintain long-term follow-up with their patients who have metastatic disease. Patchell et al. demonstrated actuarial recurrence rates exceeding 80% after whole-brain radiotherapy (36 Gy in 12 fractions) for solitary brain metastasis (20). It is therefore clear that conventional fractionated whole-brain radiotherapy by itself is inadequate for a substantial number of good prognosis patients (particularly in ambulatory patients with no other systemic metastases).

III. SURGICAL RESECTION

Because of the poor long-term control rates of all brain metastasis with conventional radiotherapy, resection of solitary brain metastasis has been advocated in good prognosis patients. Because of patient selection for surgery, retrospective studies of brain-metastasis patients undergoing craniotomy are difficult to interpret (5,11,12,25,28). Fortunately, randomized trials in patients with miscellaneous brain metastases have been performed by Patchell et al. and, more recently, by Noordijk et al. (19,20). Both studies documented not only superior tumor control, but also superior survival for patients undergoing surgical resection plus radiotherapy when compared to radiotherapy alone (median survivals: 40 vs. 15 weeks for the Patchell study, and 10 vs. 6 months for the Noordijk study) (19,20).

Several authors have reported on the outcome of malignant melanoma patients in particular who have undergone resection of brain metastasis. Brega et al. reported on 13 melanoma patients who underwent 19 craniotomies (5 patients needed a second operation) (5). The median survival was 10 months with no 30-day mortality. Wornom et al. reported 11% mortality and 22% morbidity in their series of 17 patients (28). Guazzo et al. reported major complications in 17% of 31 patients in their series (11). Hafstrin et al. found that 7/25 melanoma brain-metastasis patients who had craniotomy and resection died within one month: 3 from postoperative complications, 4 from tumor progression (12).

These studies indicate that the outcomes after surgical resection followed by whole-brain irradiation are better than the results after conventional radiotherapy alone. Unfortunately, surgical resection is not an option for many patients with deeply located tumors or multiple tumors, or for those with high medical risks for surgery.

IV. STEREOTACTIC RADIOSURGERY

Radiosurgery has been defined as the single-session, closed-skull destruction of a stereotactically defined intracranial target with high-dose ionizing external-beam irradiation (14). Normally, the procedure starts with placement of a stereotactic frame by a neurosurgeon. The patient can undergo stereotactic computed tomographic or magnetic resonance imaging with the frame in place to define the precise coordinates of any imaging-defined target. A customized computer-generated radiation isodose plan is then designed using techniques that allow relative sparing of radiation dose to surrounding normal tissue. The radiation is administered in a single treatment and the frame is removed. The entire procedure can usually be performed in a single morning under local anesthesia; children under 12 often require general anesthesia.

The Gamma Knife® was the first radiation device designed specifically for stereotactic radiosurgery. It uses 201 separate highly collimated cobalt 60 beams capable of accurately producing spherical radiation dose distributions with 4, 8, 14, or 18 mm collimators. Nonspherical volumetric radiation distributions are produced by computer-planned combinations of multiple isocenters. The dramatic success of Gamma Knife radiosurgery in treating arteriovenous malformations and acoustic neuromas stimulated the development of methods to imitate these radiation distributions with modified linear accelerators (Linac). Linac radiosurgery uses a single photon radiation source directed at the target with multiple arcs (17).

A. Radiosurgery Results for Metastases

There have been a number of reports on the effectiveness of radiosurgery in treating brain metastases (1,2,7–9,13,16, 18,24). The Gamma Knife Users Group series is a representative multicenter study of radiosurgery in 116 patients with solitary brain metastasis, 24% of whom had malignant melanoma (8). The median follow-up was 12 months after the diagnosis of brain metastasis and seven months after radiosurgery. In 71 patients, radiosurgery was part of the initial management, and 45 patients had radiosurgery when their brain metastases regrew after initial fractionated whole-brain radiotherapy. The median survival was 11 months from radiosurgery and 20 months after diagnosis.

Multivariate analysis of postradiosurgery survival identified histology as the only significant variable ($p = 0.041$). Survival was better for breast cancer [as in the RTOG whole brain radiotherapy study (4)] and worse for melanoma and renal cell cancer compared to other histologies. However, patients with melanoma or renal cell carcinoma had better local control compared to other histologies ($p = 0.0006$), with no failures recorded at the time of data analysis. The overall actuarial tumor control rate was 85% at two years. Univariate and multivariate analyses identified significantly improved tumor control in patients who received radiosurgery and whole-brain radiotherapy compared to radiosurgery alone ($p = 0.011$). From this data, radiosurgery proved highly effective treatment for the brain tumor, but survival in the various histotypes of cancer was limited by systemic disease. Two-year actuarial rates for developing radiation necrosis requiring surgical resection and for symptomatic edema were 4% and 11% respectively. The two-year actuarial rate of tumor hemorrhage after radiosurgery was 8%.

Alexander et al. recently reported their results in 248 patients who had 421 brain metastases treated with linac radiosurgery from 1986–1993 at the Harvard Joint Center for Radiation Therapy (1). Their median follow up was 36 months. Solitary metastases were treated in 177 patients. Two metastases were treated by radiosurgery in 52 patients, and three or more metastases in 19 patients. Radiosurgery was used in 60 patients as an initial boost treatment (with fractionated whole-brain irradiation) and in 188 patients for recurrent tumors. In 77 patients, no systemic extracranial metastases were present, and 171 were classified as having stable extracranial metastases. Relatively radioresistant tumors (melanoma, renal cell carcinoma, or sarcoma) were treated in 30% of the patients. The median minimum tumor dose for radiosurgery (Dmin) was 15 Gy. The median target volume was 3 cc. Multivariate analysis revealed that survival was associated significantly with the lack of any active systemic disease and age less than sixty. The actuarial tumor control rates were similar to the Gamma Knife Users Group study (85% at one year and 65% at two years). Multivariate analysis of local failure found it to be significantly elevated in patients with recurrent tumors (compared to those treated at presentation) and tumors with infratentorial locations. They did not find any significant association with histology. Their higher local failure rate with infratentorial tumors may be related to inadequate CT imaging of the posterior fossa from bone artifacts. Complications were limited to mass effect requiring surgery in 7% of patients and the development of cranial neuropathies in 1% of patients.

B.   Comparison of Surgical Resection and Radiosurgery

Auchter et al. recently reported a comparison of the effectiveness of surgical resection and radiosurgery for solitary brain metastasis (2). They compiled a multi-institutional series of patients with potentially resectable solitary brain metastasis who were initially managed with radiosurgery. The authors present a strong case for replacing surgical resection with radiosurgery as the treatment of choice for managing solitary brain metastasis. Their series of patients with resectable brain metastasis is comparable to the patients in the randomized trials of Patchell et al. and Noordijk et al. that showed the superiority of surgical resection followed by whole-brain radiotherapy over WB-XRT alone (19,20). Auchter's series includes 122 patients who met their entry criteria (solitary metastasis by CT or MR with documented extracranial cancer; surgically resectable metastasis; no prior brain XRT or brain surgery; histology that is not small cell, lymphoma, or germ cell; no urgent need for surgery; Karnofsky performance status (KPS) > 70%, and age > 18). Median follow-up was 123 weeks. The overall initial response rate was 59% (25% complete, 34% partial). Stable disease was seen in 36% and progressive disease in 6%. In-field recurrence developed in 14% and intracranial out-of-radiosurgery-field relapse in 22%. Median survival was 56 weeks, with 25% of the deaths from CNS progression. Multivariate analysis identified the presence of extracranial metastases and poor KPS score to be related to decreased survival (but not age or histology).

Figure 1 compares median overall survival and survival with KPS ≥ 70% (independent function) for the whole-brain radiotherapy (WB-XRT) and surgery groups from the randomized trials of Patchell and Noordijk to those reported by Auchter, et al. (2,19,20). Both overall and independent median survivals were better than the WB-XRT and surgery arms of both studies. Local control also is favorable for the radiosurgery study (14%), compared to both the surgery arm (20%) and WB-XRT arm (52%) of Patchell's study.

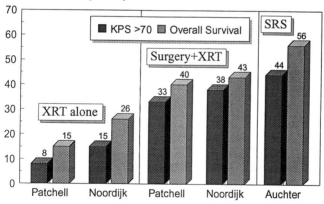

FIGURE 1 Median independent survival (KPS functional score of 70 or greater) and median overall survival for patients with resectable solitary brain metastasis treated in the whole-brain radiotherapy (XRT) and surgical resection plus XRT arms from the randomized trials of Patchell et al. (Ref. 20) and Noordijk et al. (Ref. 19), compared to the matched series of patients undergoing stereotactic radiosurgery (SRS) in the multi-institutional series of Auchter et al. (Ref. 2).

Between Auchter's series and the other published results of radiosurgery, which also include unresectable brain metastases, it is safe to conclude that radiosurgery is at least equally effective for most patients and may be superior in some.

Rutigliano et al. recently published an extensive cost–benefit comparison of gamma knife radiosurgery and surgical resection for solitary brain metastasis (23). The report concluded that radiosurgery had a lower uncomplicated procedure cost, a lower average complications cost per case, a lower total cost per procedure; and that radiosurgery was more effective and had a better incremental cost effectiveness per life-year. Treatment-related morbidity and mortality were higher for surgery (30% and 7% respectively) than they were for radiosurgery (4% and 0%).

C. Radiosurgery of Malignant Melanoma

The University of Pittsburgh experience with Gamma Knife radiosurgery of brain metastasis from malignant melanoma was first reported by Somaza et al (26). From May 1988 to May 1992, 23 melanoma patients with 32 brain metastases were managed with radiosurgery. Median follow-up was 12 months (range: 3–38 months). Solitary metastases were treated in 19 patients (4 in the brainstem). Multiple metastases were treated in 4 patients (two patients had brainstem lesions treated). The mean KPS score was 85% (range: 50–90%). Recurrent tumors were treated in four patients 3 to 12 months after initial whole-brain radiotherapy. Intratumoral hemorrhage was identified prior to radiosurgery in eight patients. Perioperative corticosteroids were used in 15 patients believed to have symptomatic peritumoral edema. Out of the 21 patients with documented extracranial metastases, 11 received chemotherapy (7 before and 4 after radiosurgery) and seven underwent immunotherapy (4 before and 3 after radiosurgery).

Tumor growth after radiosurgery was not identified in any patient, although one patient required a surgical resection one month after radiosurgery for tumor hemorrhage (giving a local control rate of 31/32 or 97%). Tumors regressed in 13/32 (41%) and peritumoral edema decreased in 9/15 (60%). Figure 2 shows a typical response. Two patients developed metastases elsewhere in the brain. Eight of 15 patients with pretreatment neurological deficits had evidence of improvement after radiosurgery. There was no treatment-related mortality, and morbidity was limited to 3/23 patients with perioperative nausea, emesis, and/or dizziness. Figure 3 shows survival after diagnosis of brain metastasis (median 9 months) and after radiosurgery (median 7 months). We have

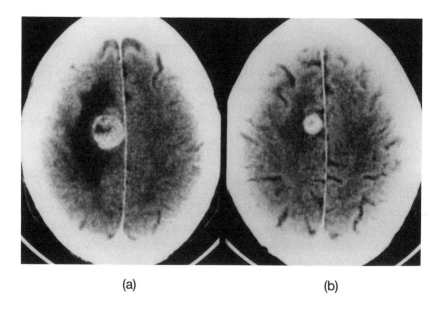

(a)   (b)

FIGURE 2 Posterior frontal lobe metastasis from malignant melanoma at (a) the time of radiosurgery and (b) four months after 30 Gy of whole brain radiotherapy and gamma knife radiosurgery to 16 Gy minimum tumor dose, 32 Gy maximum dose.

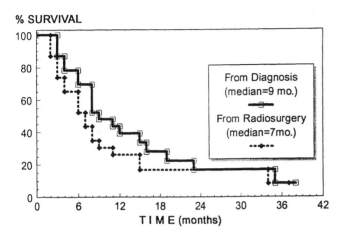

FIGURE 3 Survival from diagnosis and from radiosurgery in 23 patients with brain metastasis from malignant melanoma. (From Ref. 26.)

now managed 60 patients with melanoma brain metastasis using Gamma Knife radiosurgery as part of our overall experience in the first 2000 patients.

V. MANAGEMENT STRATEGIES

There are several different strategies that can be utilized for melanoma brain metastasis. Patients with small (3 cm diameter or less) solitary brain metastases are reasonable candidates for either radiosurgery alone or radiosurgery combined with WB-XRT if they have a good prognosis (no known extracranial systemic disease and good functional status). Radiosurgery alone (without whole-brain radiotherapy) can spare patients side effects at the expense of relapse elsewhere in the brain (9,13,15). Patients with large (3 cm or more in diameter) brain metastases who have an otherwise relatively good prognosis, especially with symptoms from mass effect unrelieved by corticosteroids, are better candidates for surgical resection than radiosurgery.

The guidelines are unclear for when radiosurgery should be used in patients with solitary brain metastases at presentation (with or without WB-XRT), versus treating with WB-XRT alone initially and reserving radiosurgery for salvage therapy. Most physicians would agree that the latter approach, of withholding aggressive local therapy like radiosurgery or surgical resection, is too conservative for young patients with no other systemic disease. Such an approach may be appropriate in older patients with poor functional status and systemic disease progression in the face of systemic therapy (1,2,16,18).

The use of radiosurgery as part of the initial management of patients with multiple metastases is another controversial issue. Data from autopsy studies, as well as the high local control rates that have been achieved in patients with two, three, and even more metastases after either surgical resection or radiosurgery, challenge the conventional wisdom that patients with more than one brain metastasis are likely to have tumor seeding throughout the brain (1,3,21). The vast majority of these patients seem to have only limited numbers of brain metastases over time (1,3,21). The role of aggressive management in patients with multiple brain metastasis is being investigated in a University of Pittsburgh Phase III clinical trial for patients with 2–4 metastases (from melanoma or other sites). All patients receive whole-brain XRT to 30 Gy/12 fractions and then are randomized to receive either immediate radiosurgery or a plan to use radiosurgery as a salvage treatment.

The effectiveness and safety of stereotactic radiosurgery for melanoma brain metastasis is well documented. Whereas brain disease used to spell disaster for most patients, an effective therapy is now available that puts additional pressure on physicians and scientists to manage the complex spectrum of systemic disease that these longer-surviving patients now present.

REFERENCES

1. Alexander E, Moriarty TM, Davis RB, Wen PY, Fine HA, Black PM, Kooy HM, Loeffler JS. Stereotactic radiosurgery for the definitive, noninvasive treatment of brain metastases. JNCI 1995; 87:34–40.

2. Auchter RM, Lamond JP, Alexander EA, Buatti JM, Chappell R, Friedman WA, Kinsella TJ, Levin AB, Noyes WR, Schultz CJ, Loeffler JS, Mehta MP. A multi-institutional outcome and prognostic factor analysis of radiosurgery for resectable single brain metastasis. Int J Radiat Oncol Biol Phys 1996; 35: (in press).

3. Bindal RK, Sawaya R, Leavens ME, et al. Surgical treatment of multiple brain metastases. J Neurosurg 1993; 79:210–216.

4. Borgelt B, Gelber R, Kramer S, Brady L, Chang C, Davis L, Perez C, Hendrickson F. The palliation of brain metastases: The final results of the first two studies by the radiation therapy oncology group. Int J Radiat Oncol Biol Phys 1980; 6:1–9.

5. Brega K, Robinson W, Winston K, et al. Surgical resection of brain metastases in malignant melanoma. Cancer 1990; 66: 2105–2110.

6. Budman DR, Camacho E, Wittes RE. The current causes of death in patients with malignant melanoma. Cancer 1978; 14:327–330.

7. Engenhart R, Kimmig BN, Hover KH, et al. Long-term follow-up for brain metastases treated by percutaneous stereotactic single high-dose irradiation. Cancer 1993; 71(4):1353–1361.

8. Flickinger JC, Kondziolka D, Lunsford LD, et al. A multi-institutional experience with stereotactic radiosurgery for solitary brain metastasis. Int J Radiat Oncol Biol Phys 1994; 28(4): 797–802.

9. Fuller BG, Kaplan ID, Adler, J, et al. Stereotaxic radiosurgery for brain metastases: the importance of adjuvant whole brain irradiation. Int J Radiat Oncol Biol Phys 1992; 23:413–418.

10. Gelber R, Larson M, Borget BB, Kramer S. Equivalence of radiation schedules for the palliative treatment of brain metastases in patients with favorable prognosis. Cancer 1981; 48: 1749–1753.

11. Guazzo EP, Atkinson L, Weidmann M, et al. Management of solitary melanoma metastasis of the brain. Aust NZ J Surg 1989; 59:321–324.
12. Hafstrin L, Jonsson PE, Stromblad LG. Intracranial metastasis of malignant melanoma treated by surgery. Cancer 1980; 46:208–2090.
13. Kihlstrom L, Karlsson B, Lindquist C. Gamma knife surgery for cerebral metastasis: Implications for survival based on 16 years experience. Ster & Func Neurosurg 61(Suppl) 1993; 1: 45–50.
14. Leksell L. The stereotaxic method and radiosurgery of the brain. Acta Chir Scand 1951; 102:316–319.
15. Lishner M, Feld R, Payne DG, et al. Late neurological complications after prophylactic cranial irradiation in patients with small-cell lung cancer: The Toronto experience. J Clin Oncol 1990; 8:215–221.
16. Loeffler JS, Shrieve DC. What is appropriate therapy for a patient with a single brain metastasis? Int J Radiat Oncol Biol Phys 1994; 29(4):915–917.
17. Lutz W, Winston KR, Maleki PV. A system for stereotactic radiosurgery with a linear accelerator. Int J Radiat Oncol Biol Phys 1988; 14:373–381.
18. Mehta MP, Rozental JM, Levin AB, et al. Defining the role of radiosurgery in the management of brain metastases. Int J Radiat Oncol Biol Phys 1992; 24(4):619–25.
19. Noordijk EM, Vecht CJ, Haaxma-Reiche H, et al. The choice of treatment of single brain metastasis should be based on extracranial tumor activity and age. Int J Radiat Biol Phys 1994; 29:711–717.
20. Patchell RA, Tibbs PA, Walsh JW, et al. A randomized trial of surgery in the treatment of single metastases to the brain. NEJM 1990; 322:494.
21. Pickren JW, Lopez G, Tzukada Y, Lane WW: Brain metastases. An autopsy study. Cancer Treat Symp 1983; 2:295–313.
22. Restas S, Gershny AR. Central nervous system involvement in malignant melanoma. Cancer 1988; 61:1926–1934.
23. Rutigliano MJ, Lunsford LD, Kondziolka D, Strauss MJ, Khanna V, Green M: The cost effectiveness of stereotactic radiosurgery versus surgical resection in the treatment of

solitary metastatic brain tumors. Neurosurg 1995; 37: 445–455.

24. Shaw E, Farnan N, Souhami L, Dinapoli R, Kline R, Loeffler J, Fisher B. Radiosurgical treatment of previously irradiated primary brain tumors and brain metastasis: Final report of radiation oncology group (RTOG) protocol 90-05. Int J Radiat Oncol Biol Phys 1995; 32(S1):145

25. Smalley SR, Laws ER, O'Fallon JR, Shaw EG, Schray MF. Resection for solitary brain metastasis: Role of adjuvant radiation and prognostic variables in 229 patients. J Neurosurg 1992; 77:531–540.

26. Somaza S, Kondziolka D, Lunsford LD, Kirkwood J, Flickinger J. Stereotactic radiosurgery for cerebral metastatic melanoma. J Neurosurg 1993; 79:661–666.

27. Vlock DR, Kirkwood JM, Leutzinger C, Kapp DS, Fischer JJ. High dose fraction radiation therapy for intracranial metastases of malignant melanoma. Cancer 1982; 49:2289–2294.

28. Wornom IL, Soong SJ, Urist MM, et al. Surgical palliative treatment for distant metastases of melanoma. Ann Surg 1986; 204:181–185.

11

PCR-Based Detection of Malignant Cells
Toward Molecular Staging?

Ulrich Keilholz and Martina Willhauck
University of Heidelberg
Heidelberg, Germany

I. INTRODUCTION

It is the current understanding of the process of metastasis that single neoplastic cells leave the primary tumor and travel to distant body sites via the lymphatic system and the bloodstream. If single neoplastic cells or small aggregates travel via the lymphatics, they may find a suitable environment for survival and possibly expansion and further spread in the first draining lymph node, which has been designated as *sentinal lymph node*. If the tumor cells spread hematogenously, multiple factors will determine the organ site, where they may survive and possibly give rise to further metastases. Many details of this process, especially the kinetics, are still under investigation, but it has always been a desire for oncologists to monitor lymphatic and hematogenous spread of neoplastic cells. Single tumor cells, in the bone marrow for example, can be detected by immunohistologic techniques; however, this method is not sufficiently sensitive to monitor reliably the process of early metastasis or minimal residual disease. Recently, PCR-based (polymerase chain reaction) methods to detect single neoplastic cells have been developed (see Table 1).

Immunohistologic investigations are based on identification of tumor-specific or tumor-associated proteins with highly specific monoclonal antibodies. Several studies confirmed that single tumor cells can be present in regional lymph nodes which appear free of tumor by macroscopical and routine light microscopical evaluation. Furthermore, single tumor cells could be detected in a proportion of patients with colon carcinoma, carcinoma of the breast, and sarcoma in the bone marrow and, occasionally, in the peripheral blood using immunohistologic techniques (1–5).

TABLE 1
Limit of Detection for Tumor Cells in Peripheral Blood and Bone Marrow

Technique	Limit of detection
Light microscopy	1 tumor cell in 100–1000 normal cells
Immunocytology	1 tumor cell in 10^5–10^6 normal cells
PCR	1 tumor cell in 10^7–10^8 normal cells

This has been suggested to be of prognostic value. Limitations of this technique are that tumor cells can be detected only if the expression of the target protein is sufficiently high, and that only a rather small proportion of a clinical sample (especially of a tissue biopsy) can be investigated with reasonable effort.

PCR-based techniques allow exponential amplification of specific regions of DNA or RNA molecules using repeated cycles of denaturation, annealing, and extension. The specifity is achieved by designing oligonucleotide primers with nucleotide sequences specific for the gene of interest. With this technique, the presence of genetic abnormalities or the expression of tumor-specific or tumor-associated genes can be utilized to detect tumor cells in a clinical specimen with highest sensitivity. By extracting the total genomic DNA or RNA from a clinical sample, PCR-based analysis offers the theoretical possibility of evaluating the whole sample in a single reaction. Over the past five years, suitable PCR assays have been developed for various types of neoplastic cells, and initial results describing the possible clinical usefulness have accumulated. This chapter summarizes the principles of PCR-based detection of occult tumor cells, as well as the currently available clinical data.

II. PRINCIPAL METHODS OF PCR ASSAYS

Prerequisites for detection of tumor cells are well-characterized structural or mutational DNA abnormalities or consistently expressed RNA sequences of tumor-associated antigens.

Genomic DNA level: Structural abnormalities (translocations, deletions, insertions), as well as specific point mutations in proto-oncogenes, represent specific alterations present in the DNA of all tumor cells, but not in normal cells of the organism, with a few possible exceptions. The most important advantages of DNA techniques are robust extraction methods from all kinds of clinical material, including paraffin embedded tissue, easy handling of DNA, and the independence of the transcriptional activity of the tumor cells. One possible disadvantage for sensitivity is that one tumor cell usually contains only a single copy of the gene of interest. The molecular abnormalities of tumor cells detectable by DNA techniques can also be determined on the RNA level, which may improve sensitivity.

RNA level: The major application of RNA techniques is the investigation of tissue-specific antigens (differentiation antigens) which are expressed only in tumor cells or in the cell-type giving rise to the malignant cell. The prerequisite is that the target gene should be expressed exclusively by tumor cells in the tissue studied, and that the normal counterparts are not present in this tissue. By carefully choosing target genes, this can be accomplished for detection of almost all solid malignancies in the peripheral blood and, possibly, in the bone marrow.

RNA-based methods require active transcription of the gene of interest but therefore have the advantage that only viable cells are detected, and usually a high copy number of the gene of interest is present in a single tumor cell. The number of copies in a tumor cell may, however, vary during the life cycle of a cell or as a result of de-differentiation.

A. DNA Amplification

In case of a tumor-specific translocation, two gene fragments are joined to a new gene, which commonly leads either to the activation of a proto-oncogene or the inactivation of a so-called tumor-suppressor gene. By choosing a pair of primers consisting of one primer for each partner of the fusion gene, a DNA fragment can be amplified that is specific for all of the particular neoplastic cells (see Figure 1). In

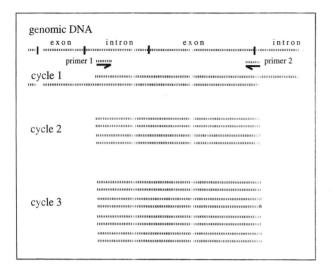

FIGURE 1 DNA PCR. 1 pair of primers (primer 1 and primer 2) are synthesized matching sequences of the gene of interest. For DNA amplification, any position of the genomic DNA can be used, regardless of whether the sequence is a coding sequence (EXON) of an intron. Primer 1 is synthesized in sense direction and primer 2 in antisense direction. During the first cycle of PCR, both primers bind to a template and a complementary strand is synthesized. Because primers usually do not bind to the same template, the synthesis does not end at the theoretical position of the second primer. After denaturation, the primers again bind to the designated site of the product from the first cycle, and, in most instances, the PCR product is now trimmed to the designated size consisting of the primer sequence on both ends and the sequence of the gene of interest in between. During subsequent cycles, the amount of PCR product increases exponentially as long as sufficient amounts of primers and nucleotides are present and the polymerase maintains full activity. If, due to repeated heating, the polymerase loses activity or primer concentration or nucleotide concentration decreases significantly, the efficiency of the PCR amplification decreases and the amount of newly synthesized PCR product reaches a plateau phase. This occurs usually after 25 to 35 cycles of PCR.

the case of B- or T-cell malignancies, the rearranged immunoglobulin or T-cell-receptor gene can also be utilized for this purpose, if the hypervariable region (CDR3-region) has been sequenced and at least one primer is located in the CDR3-region of the respective immunoglobulin or T-cell-receptor gene, or consensus primers flanking the CDR3-region can be used.

DNA amplification has been utilized for detection of minimal residual disease in hematologic malignancies such as lymphoma, in which the tumor cells have clonally rearranged immunoglobulin genes or T-cell-receptor genes or specific chromosomal translocations, such as the frequent t(14;18) translocation, as well as for CML, where a fragment of the bcr/abl-fusion gene (Philadelphia chromosome) is amplified. For solid tumors, not many specific and frequent translocations or mutations have been described so far, the best known exception being mutations of the ras proto-oncogene, where specific mutations are frequently found, especially in gastrointestinal carcinomas.

B. RNA Amplification

For detection of the vast majority of solid tumors, genes encoding for tissue-specific proteins are utilized. The most commonly used examples are summarized in Table 2. These genes are not actively transcribed in normal cells of the peripheral blood and bone marrow and probably not in lymphatic tissue; and the non-neoplastic tissue-specific cells are not present outside of their organ environment.

Some of these genes are expressed in tumor cells at a high level, whereas they are expressed at a very low level, or are undetectable, in their normal counterparts, e.g., the genes encoding for oncofetal proteins such as CEA and AFP. For genes encoding for proteins of functional importance for the normal cells, the level of expression in tumor cells may be

TABLE 2

Genes Utilized for Detection of Tumor Cells

Tumor type	Target gene
Melanoma	Tyrosinase, p97, MUCI8, MAGE-3
Prostate cancer	PSA, PSM
Gastrointestinal cancer	
stomach	CEA
pancreas	Mutated K-ras
colorectal	CEA, CK 20, mutated K-ras
Breast carcinoma	CK19, CK2, CEA
Neuroblastoma	Tyrosin-hydroxylase, N-CAM, PGP 9.5, MAGE
head and neck carcinoma	Mutated p53
Ewing's sarcoma	t(11;22)(q24;q12)
Hepatocellular carcinoma	AFP
Lung cancer	NSE, bombesin

in the same range, but may also be much lower as a consequence of de-differentiation or selection during tumor progression. An ideal marker gene would be of essential importance for survival of the neoplastic cell; however, none of the genes listed in Table 2 fits into this theoretically desirable category.

1. Method of Reverse Transcription PCR (RT-PCR)

The RNA is first extracted from the sample and reversely transcribed into cDNA (see Figure 2). Numerous protocols are available for this procedure. It has to be kept in mind that the cDNA mostly is contaminated with varying amounts of genomic DNA. The gene of interest is then amplified using specific primers. Ideally, these primers should not amplify genomic DNA. This can be achieved if one primer spans an in-

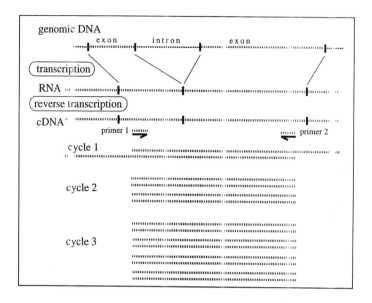

FIGURE 2 Reverse transcription PCR. In viable cells, genomic DNA is transcribed into RNA. During this process, introns are spliced and the resulting RNA strand consists only of the exon sequence. Prior to PCR amplification, the RNA has to be reversely transcribed into complementary DNA (cDNA) by an enzyme called reverse transcriptase. The resulting cDNA has a complementary sequence to the RNA and differs from the genomic DNA because of the absence of introns. After reverse transcription, the process of PCR is identical to the process of DNA amplification described in Fig. 1. If the primer sequence is chosen to match an exon sequence, both the genomic DNA and the cDNA will be amplified. The resulting PCR product of the genomic DNA is larger if an intron is present between two exons. The size difference can be used to discriminate between genomic DNA and cDNA. Alternatively, the primer sequence can span an intron. In the latter case, genomic DNA will not be amplified. For detection of occult tumor cells, it is essential to discriminate between genomic DNA and cDNA, since genomic DNA is present in any cell, but the cDNA, as a result of reverse transcription, is obtained only from viable cells actively transcribing the gene of interest.

tron of the genomic DNA which is deleted during RNA transcription. Alternatively, an intron should be in between the sequence amplified by a pair of primers, because the resulting PCR product would contain the intron if genomic DNA is amplified, facilitating easy differentiation of PCR products derived from genomic DNA and cDNA based on the size of the product.

To increase sensitivity, a second round of PCR can be performed (nested PCR) using primers for internal sequences of the PCR product generated in the first round of PCR. Besides increased sensitivity, the nested PCR also has increased specificity, because a nonspecific product generated during the first round of PCR will not be amplified further in the second round.

After PCR amplification, the product usually is detected on an agarose gel or specifically hybridized after southern blotting. In addition, the PCR product can be sequenced to verify concordance of the sequence of the PCR product with the gene of interest.

2. Sample Preparation for RT-PCR

RNA is transcribed from DNA only in viable cells. In case of disruption of the integrity of the cell, ubiquitous RNAses rapidly degrade any RNA. For these reasons, rapid processing of the clinical samples is of crucial importance and certain general precautions need to be maintained.

Tissue samples should be frozen in liquid nitrogen as soon as possible and minced frozen. The disintegrated sample is then admixed with RNA extraction buffer. Bone marrow and blood samples can be admixed directly with RNA extraction buffer, which inhibits RNAses. Prolonged storage of blood samples is to be avoided.

The lysis of erythrocytes using lysis buffers should be avoided, since this leads to significant release of RNAses and frequent RNA degradation. If gradient separation techniques are to be employed to separate red blood cells in peripheral blood from leucocytes, it has to be ensured that the tumor cells remain above the separation fluid. In the case of regular Ficoll with a specific gravity of 1.077 g/l, tumor cells may sediment with the granulocytes and erythrocytes. Split-sample analysis from melanoma patients have revealed that the majority of melanoma cells in the peripheral blood can only be separated from red blood cells if a separation medium of 1.09 g/l was used, which yields separation of all peripheral blood leucocytes from erythrocytes (6). But it is uncertain whether tumor cells are still trapped in the erythrocyte pellet. As a consequence of this observation, we recommend the use of whole blood samples or a separation medium of sufficient density for this assay.

3. RNA Extraction/cDNA Synthesis

Various protocols are available for extraction of RNA. Most often, guanidinium-isothiocyanate-phenol-chlorophorm–based extraction methods as first described by Chomczynski and Sacchi (7) are being employed. Alternatively, commercial kits for RNA extraction based on ionexchange columns have been used. Cesium chloride gradient separation techniques require long-term ultracentrifugation and are therefore less suited for routine analysis; however, these methods yield the purest RNA. Probably, all of these methods are suited for RNA extraction; however, the efficiency of RNA extraction from sample to sample and between methods varies considerably and is somewhat unpredictable. Therefore, the RNA yield and integrity have to be controlled for every sample.

Various protocols and reverse transcriptases are in use for cDNA synthesis, and most protocols yield sufficient results.

4. Polymerase Chain Reaction

Several different DNA polymerases are available. For all primers and enzymes, the optimal PCR conditions have to be established. With reliable thermal cyclers the intra- and interassay-variations of the efficiency of PCR are considerably smaller than the variations in efficiency of RNA extraction and cDNA synthesis.

III. QUALITY ASSURANCE

Figure 3a depicts all standard controls. These are routinely used to ensure accuracy of each step from RNA extraction to visualization of the PCR product.

The RNA yield can be determined photometrically at a wavelength of 260 nm; however, contaminating DNA and proteins can lead to falsely high RNA quantities. The RNA purity can be assessed using an ethidium bromide-stained MOPS agarose gel, which also allows for an assessment of relative quantity and the detection of significant degradation.

A problem is that the cDNA can not be seen directly, therefore indirect methods are necessary to verify its integrity. This is usually accomplished by PCR amplification of a housekeeping gene, such as β-2 microglobulin, β-actin, or GAPDH. The value of this assessment for efficiency of reverse transcription should not be overestimated. Housekeeping genes are expressed so abundantly that they are detected even in cDNAs of insufficient quality for reliable detection of a gene of interest at an adequate copy number. This problem can be reduced by limiting the amplification of the housekeeping gene to a number of cycles, where the PCR is still in the exponential phase (approximately 18–20 cycles for tumor tissue and cell lines, and up to 26 cycles for peripheral blood). Under these circumstances, the quality of cDNA can be assessed semiquantitatively using a 2% agarose gel.

A system to control the whole process in a single step would be desirable (see Figure 3b). One proposal is the following (see Figure 3c): A small number of cells expressing a gene that is not usually present in the sample is admixed

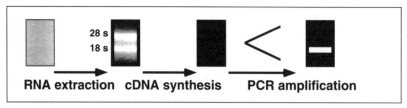

Controls (standard)

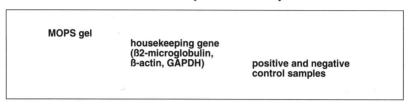

(a)

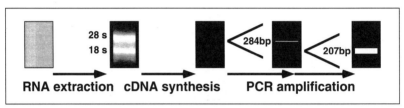

Controls (desired)

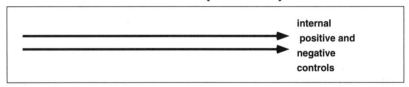

(b)

FIGURE 3 (a) After extraction of total RNA from a homogenized sample, the extract can be run on a MOPS agarose gel stained with ethidium bromide. The 28s and 18s ribosomal RNA (rRNA) bands indicate the amount of intact RNA. The amount can be quantified photometrically. The subsequent cDNA synthesis cannot be controlled directly. To determine whether amplifiable cDNA has been synthesized, a "housekeeping gene," translated in every viable cell, can be amplified by PCR and detected. If, with a limited number of PCR cycles (usually between 20 and 26), no signal is visible for the housekeeping gene, the cDNA is of insufficient quality for analysis. After

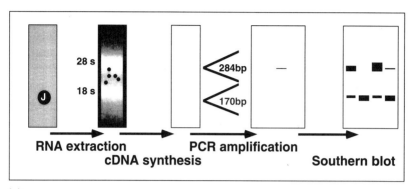

(c)

with the sample prior to processing. The copy number of the control gene should be in the same order of magnitude as the expected copy number of the gene of interest in the tumor cells (e.g., 100–1,000 cells per sample). The control gene is then carried throughout the whole process and coamplified with the tumor-cell gene in the PCR. The primers have to be designated such that the PCR product from the control gene is approximately 100 bases smaller or larger than that of the

---

PCR amplification (single round or nested PCR amplification), the PCR product can be run on an agarose gel and seen by means of ethidium bromide staining. Simultaneously processed positive and negative control samples can exclude contamination of the reagents (but not sporadic contamination) and give an estimate of the PCR sensitivity. (b) Since many problems can occur during the three-step procedure, negative and internal positive controls are desirable to control the entire process. (c) One suggestion for an internal control is to add a limited number of control cells expressing a specific gene directly to the sample. The gene product is carried through the whole procedure and can simultaneously be amplified in the PCR reaction with the gene of interest providing an internal sensitivity control. When establishing such a system, competition between the PCR of the gene of interest and the control gene has to be excluded.

PCR product from the gene specific for the tumor cell. For this assay, significant primer competition has to be excluded. If 30 cycles of PCR are employed followed by subsequent southern blotting and specific hybridization of the tumor cell gene and the control gene, the PCR product for the control gene should be clearly visible for every sample, as long as every step was performed with sufficient efficacy.

As a simultaneous negative control, the sample should be processed in duplicate but in the absence of reverse transcriptase in one of the duplicates. Thus, in the second sample, no RNA is transcribed to cDNA, and a positive result would indicate contamination.

The importance of positive and negative controls for the PCR assay cannot be overemphasized (6,8–11). Before widespread and possibly commercial application may begin, it is of crucial importance to establish very rigid quality-assurance systems. Otherwise, it will not be possible to compare results of different groups and establish the usefulness of this method in the clinical setting. Figure 4 summarizes a setting of positive and negative controls ensuring the detection of systematic and sporadic contamination and differences in sensitivity.

IV. SURVEY OF CLINICAL DATA

For most of the solid malignancies, the expression of tissue-specific genes has been utilized for detection of occult disease (see Table 2). In contrast, defined genetic abnormalities are most often used for the monitoring of minimal residual disease in lymphomas and leukemias, which is not described in this chapter.

A. Melanoma

A number of specific genes encoding for melanosomal proteins are selectively expressed in melanocytes and melanomas. Ty-

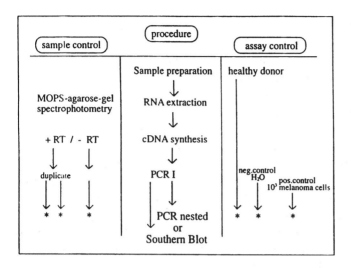

FIGURE 4 A set of controls for diagnostic PCR. Contamination and low sensitivity can result from any step of the process of sample preparation, RNA extraction, cDNA synthesis, and PCR (center lane). For detection of tumor cells in a series of patient samples, the amount of RNA should be estimated by MOPS agarose gel or spectrophotometry. The cDNA synthesis should be performed in parallel with and without reverse transcriptase. In the sample without reverse transcriptase, no cDNA is synthesized; if there is a PCR product, then contamination has occurred. For the sample where the reverse transcriptase had been added, the resulting cDNA is subjected in duplicate to PCR amplification. The duplicate samples should reveal identical results. To assure the reliability of the whole assay (right lane), at least one sample from a healthy donor should be analyzed in parallel to a series of patient samples. For the PCR, a negative water control is suitable to rule out systematic contamination of reagents, and a positive control of a cDNA from a sample with a low number ($10^2–10^3$) of tumor cells should reveal a positive PCR result, if the PCR is of sufficient efficiency.

rosinase is the first enzyme of the melanin biosynthesis, a monooxygenase catalyzing the conversion of tyrosine to dopa and of dopa to dopaquinone. Tyrosinase is therefore one of the most specific markers of melanocytes and conserved in a proportion of albinos as well as in most amelanotic melanoma metastases. The expression of the tyrosinase gene is most widely used for the detection of circulating melanoma cells. Further melanocyte-specific proteins include gp100, which is recognized by the diagnostic antibodies HMB45 and NKI-beteb (12), Melan-A/MART1 (13,14), and a family of tyrosinase-related proteins. GP100 is less suited for monitoring of melanoma since it is known to be lost during tumor progression (15,16). The expression of Melan-A/MART1 and tyrosinase-related protein are less well studied, but it was shown that they are also lost in a significant percentage of metastatic lesions as detected by specific monoclonal antibodies (17,18). Melanomas also express tumor-associated genes such as the MAGE family: about 60% of metastatic lesions are positive for MAGE-1, and 80% for MAGE-3, as detected by PCR (19–22).

In 1991, Smith et al. (23) reported that circulating melanoma cells can be detected by PCR amplification of tyrosinase RNA. They developed a PCR assay, which is still used frequently today because of the optimal primer design (see Figure 5). The primers, designated as HTYR1 to HTYR4, exploit the presence of two introns in the tyrosinase gene. HTYR1 spans one intron, and a second intron is located in between the nested primers HTYR3 and 4. This primer design virtually excludes amplification of genomic DNA.

The initial report led to a number of more detailed investigations regarding the presence of tyrosinase RNA in peripheral blood of melanoma patients (24–30). Nonmelanoma controls were always negative for expression of tyrosinase, suggesting that normal melanocytes do not circulate in blood, and that the presence of tyrosinase RNA can be judged as evidence for circulating melanoma cells. Hoon et al. described a multiple marker PCR (28) where no false-positives occurred,

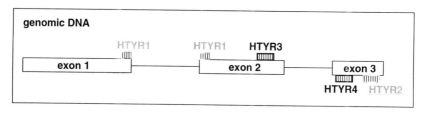

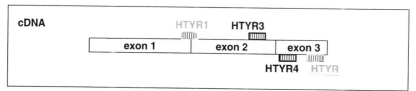

FIGURE 5 Primer design for amplification of human tyrosinase with nested PCR. The primers HTYR 1 and HTYR 2 have been designed for the first round of PCR. Amplification of genomic DNA is excluded because HTYR 1 spans an intron. The primer pair HTYR 3 and HTYR 4 for the nested PCR amplify a region of the gene where, in the genomic DNA, another intron would be amplified, resulting in a larger PCR product than that from correctly spliced RNA. (From Ref. 21.)

except for two healthy controls expressing the MUC18 gene (which is not specific for melanoma).

Subsequent investigations attempted to quantify the tyrosinase expression using two different approaches. Curry et al. (31) developed a competetive PCR assay with a heterologous DNA (PCR MIMIC, Figure 6). Brossart et al. (32) used Southern blotting of the PCR product and standardization, to the expression of a housekeeping gene (see Figure 7). For the first approach, several PCR-reactions per sample are necessary, but it yields true quantitative PCR results. In the second approach, the PCR assay is semiquantitative, but the comparison with a housekeeping gene corrects for the sometimes considerable differences in efficacy of RNA extraction and cDNA synthesis.

The results reported in melanoma patients vary considerably among different laboratories. This is most obvious in

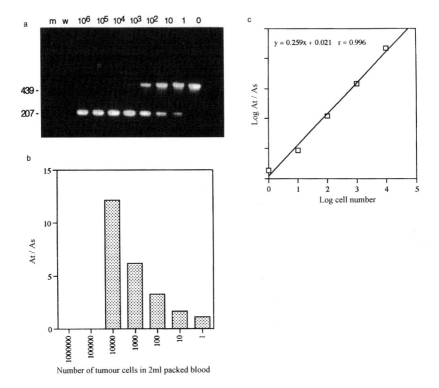

FIGURE 6 Use of competitive PCR to quantify a tenfold dilution of MM200 melanoma cells. (From Ref. 31.) (a) PRC products were run on an ethidium bromide stained agarose gel. Lane 1: DNA size markers; lane 2: water control; lanes 3 to 9: cDNA from 10^6 to 1 melanoma cells amplified in the presence of two times 10^{-5} atomoles of tyrosinase mimic; lane 10: no target cDNA. (b) After densitometric scanning of the gel, the ratio of amplified products—the RT/AS ratio—was blotted against the appropriate dilution of melanoma cells. (c) The log of RT/AS blotted against the log of the cull number reveals a linear relation.

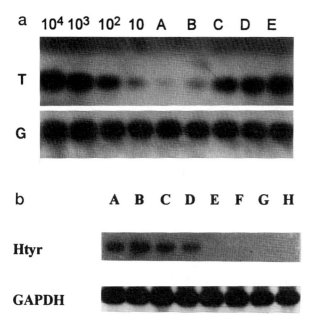

FIGURE 7 Quantitative detection of tyrosinase transcripts. (a) Southern blot analysis of PCR-amplified tyrosinase (T) and GAPDH (G) expression in serially diluted SK Mel 28 cells (10–10⁴) and patient samples. PCR comprises 23 cycles for GAPDH and 28 cycles for tyrosinase amplification. (b) Southern blot analysis of PCR-amplified human tyrosinase (Htyr) and GAPDH expression in patients and probands; B, patients in complete remission after cytokine treatment; C and D, patients with no evidence of disease after cytokine treatment and surgical removal of remaining tumor; E–H, healthy controls, and patients with carcinomas of the colon, lung, and breast. (From Ref. 32.)

stage IV melanoma patients, where the percentage of patients with evidence for circulating melanoma cells ranges between 23% and 100%. The most likely explanation for the discrepancy is in the methodological differences in sample processing, affecting the efficacy of RNA extraction and cDNA synthesis, which differ among laboratories, as seen in Table 3. The use of Ficoll hipaque density gradient sepa-

TABLE 3

Detection of Circulating Melanoma Cells in Patients with Distant
Metastases (Stage IV)

Reference	Sample processing	Marker gene	TYR mRNA positive samples per number of patients
23	Whole blood	Tyrosinase	4/7
24	Whole blood	Tyrosinase	21/21
27	Ficoll 1.077	Tyrosinase	25/73
29	Whole blood	Tyrosinase	0/6[a]
28	Ficoll 1.007	Multiple	46/48[b]
30	Whole blood	Tyrosinase	9/32
33	Whole blood	Tyrosinase	33/35
Own observation	Whole blood	Tyrosinase	30/35[c] 65/81

[a] Storage of blood samples without buffer at –70°C prior to processing.
[b] Two of 39 healthy control samples tested positive.
[c] Untreated patients.
[d] After treatment.

ration prior to RNA extraction, especially, may significantly decrease the number of positive results in stage IV patients. Quality assurance initiatives have been started recently in Europe and in the United States to resolve the impact of methodological differences for sensitivity and to facilitate comparison of the results from different laboratories.

The detection of circulating melanoma cells could be particularly useful in treating earlier stages of the disease and, theoretically, could guide decisions concerning adjuvant treatment strategies. To date, the percentage of patients with stages I, II, and III melanoma and PCR evidence for circulating melanoma cells varies considerably in different reports, which may not only be a result of methodological differences but also of differences in patient selection. Two analyses, however, already suggest that the PCR result is of prognostic value in melanoma: Battayani and colleagues (27) described that, after resection of regional lymph node metastasis, the likelihood of recurrence within four months was significantly higher in patients with a positive tyrosinase signal; and that patients with stage IV disease and a positive signal were significantly more likely to experience rapid disease progression within four months as compared to patients who tested negative (see Table 4a and b). Mellado and colleagues (33) reported from a prospective investigation that, in stage II and III, the presence of tyrosinase transcripts in the peripheral blood was associated with significantly shorter disease-free survival. Larger prospective investigations are necessary (and currently underway)

TABLE 4a
TYR-PCR in Stage II Melanoma Prior to
Lymph Node Dissection

Development of metastases within 6 months	TYR-PCR+	TYR-PCR–	total
No recurrence	6	37	43
Recurrence	8 (57%)	7 (16%)	15 (26%)
Total	14	44	58

TABLE 4b
TYR-PCR in Melanoma Patients
with Distant Metastases

Evaluation within 4 months of PCR	TYR-PCR +	TYR-PCR –	total
Rapid progression	15 (60%)	7 (15%)	22 (30%)
Slow progression	5	20	25
Stable disease	5	21	26
Total	25	48	73

Source: Ref. 27.

in order to confirm the prognostic value of the PCR assay, especially in melanoma patients with disease stages I through III who are surgically rendered disease-free, as well as to address the value of adjuvant treatment strategies (e.g., interferon-α) in PCR-positive and -negative patients in the setting of large controlled clinical trials designed to investigate the guiding of treatment decisions based on PCR results.

In melanoma patients with stage IV disease in long-term complete remission (without clinical evidence of recurrence for more than five years) after treatment with IFN-α and IL-2, with or without resection of residual metastases, tyrosinase transcripts have been detected. Quantitative assessment revealed a very low number of tyrosinase transcripts (see Figure 8), equivalent to less than 100 SK mel 28 melanoma cells (32). It is not known whether a rise in signal intensity could be an early indicator for relapse.

The value of PCR for the examination of tissue was recently investigated. Lymph-node preparations from patients with stage I or II melanoma were analyzed pathologically and by PCR in one series (34). Thirty-eight percent of 29 regional lymph-node samples had pathologic evidence for melanoma cells, whereas 66%, including all pathologically positive nodes, were RT-PCR-positive as assessed by detection of tyrosinase RNA. The results of lymph-node investigation are very encouraging, but larger studies underlining the clinical value of this procedure are necessary (11). Furthermore, it is important to strictly avoid contact with skin when processing tissue samples to avoid contamination with melanocytes. For peripheral blood samples, contamination with skin melanocytes is less of a problem if the first syringe of blood drawn after venipuncture is discarded and another syringe is subsequently used to draw the sample for the PCR assay.

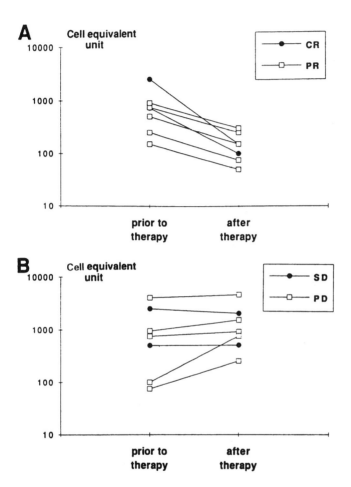

FIGURE 8 Results of quantitative assessment of tyrosinase transcripts in the peripheral blood of patients before and after cytokine treatment. The PCR product has been quantified as described in Fig. 7 and compared to serial dilutions of SK MEL 28 melanoma cells. The result is given in SK MEL 28 equivalent units. (A) Patients who responded to cytokine treatment with a partial remission. (B) Patients with stable or progressive disease after cytokine treatment.

B. Prostate Cancer

Cancer of the prostate, one of the most common malignancies in older men, has a highly variable course. It may progress and metastasize rapidly, or it may behave rather benignly, not threatening survival or impairing the quality of life. It would therefore be desirable to assess the metastatic potential early. Two marker proteins have been used for serologic screening purposes: prostate-specific antigen (PSA) and, more recently, prostate-specific membrane antigen (PSM). While PSA can be downregulated or lost during tumor progression, the expression level of PSM increases with tumor progression. Therefore, PSM is an excellent candidate gene for use in the detection of prostate cancer cells.

RT-PCR assays for both genes have been established (35–39). There were no reports of false positives from healthy controls or patients with benign prostate disease and elevated serum PSA levels. Table 5 summarizes the PCR results from different patient groups with localized or advanced prostate cancer (35–42). The assay for the expression of PSM

TABLE 5

RT-PCR for Prostate-Specific Markers in Patients
with Prostatic Cancer

| | | No. of positive samples/No. of patients | |
Reference	Target gene	Localized cancer	Distant metastases
35	PSA	4/12	—
39	PSA	5/65	1/14
37	PSA	1/33	4/24
	PSM	22/33	16/24
42	PSM	40/60	—
	PSA	20/60	—
40	PSA	4/25	25/72
41	PSA	0/7	9/18

appears to be more sensitive than that for the expression of PSA (38). The frequency of positive results for either antigen increases with stage of invasion (37). Positive PCR results have been reported by several groups in patients with distant metastases but normal serum levels of PSA or PSM protein, suggesting an increase in sensitivity of the PCR assay over serological assays. Prospective clinical investigations have to be carried out to establish the clinical usefulness of PCR results in patients with prostate cancer.

C. Gastrointestinal Cancer

Many cancers of the gastrointestinal system, such as colorectal cancer, pancreatic carcinoma, and gastric carcinoma, express the carcinoembryonic antigen (CEA). CEA is also expressed at a low level in normal gastrointestinal mucosa. The serological detection of CEA is well established as a marker useful for monitoring of patients with gastrointestinal cancers, although it is not completely specific. Several investigations have utilized the expression of CEA to detect minimal cancer (43) and suggest a correlation between PCR results and extent of disease. Other approaches are based on the finding that many gastrointestinal carcinomas are associated with specific mutations in the K-ras proto-oncogene. The specific mutation in codon 12 has been demonstrated by PCR in the stool of patients with colorectal carcinoma (44) and in the excretory product of the pancreas in patients with pancreatic cancer (45,46). Current studies are testing the usefulness of this technique for screening purposes. Cell-structure proteins, especially cytokeratins, also have been used as target genes to detect tumor cells (47). Cytokeratin 18 (CK18) has been the target protein for immunohistologic techniques, and its prognostic usefulness is well established. However, by PCR, the CK18 gene is readily detected in blood of normal individuals, probably because of the presence of pseudogenes (48). Another isoform, cytokeratin 19, has led to false-positive results if nested PCR was employed (49). CK20 seems to be more specific (47). A more recent report describes CD44 splice variants to detect colon carcinoma cells (50). Studies are necessary to investigate the value of these different approaches in the clinical setting.

D. Carcinoma of the Breast

Cytokeratins and CEAs have also been used as target genes for the detection of breast carcinoma cells (51–53). However, because of the lack of sufficiently large studies, the clinical utility of these approaches has not yet been established.

E. Neuroblastoma

Neuroblastoma, the fourth most frequent pediatric malignancy, is derived from the embryonic neural crest and possesses different features of the autonomous nervous system. Although great progress has been made in the understanding of chromosomal abnormalities, no specific structural abnormality has been defined that is suitable for the detection of circulating tumor cells. Tyrosine hydroxylase, however, is frequently expressed as a tissue-specific gene suitable for the detection of neuroblastoma cells (54–57). The percent of positive findings in bone marrow has been shown to increase with stage, reaching 100% (in a small series of 11 patients) in stage IV (57). After cytotoxic treatment, tyrosinase hydroxylase mRNA disappears from peripheral blood; but it is frequently detectable again at the time of clinical relapse, and may be an early indicator for relapse (56).

Other candidate genes include members of the MAGE family, PGP 9.5, and a rather specific isoform of the adhesion molecule N-CAM (utilizing exons 17 and 19). The investigations, however, are not conclusive, and false positives have been reported (58).

F. Carcinoma of the Head and Neck

Local recurrence of head and neck cancer occurs in up to half of patients with microscopically negative surgical margins. Mutations in the p53 gene are the most common specific genetic alterations in carcinomas of the head and neck. Brennan and colleagues have investigated the p53 tumor-suppressor gene in the resection margins in patients who appeared to have had complete tumor resection on the basis of a negative histopathological assessment (59). The p53 gene was amplified from DNA extracted from margins of the surgical resection specimen. The PCR products were then cloned into *Escherichia coli*, and the clones were hybridized with an individual probe prepared from the patients original tumor. This approach facilitated a semiquantitative assessment of the presence of p53 in the tissue sample. The presence of the tumor-specific p53 mutations in the resection margins in 13 of 25 patients was associated with a significant increase in the probability of local recurrence. This approach is labor-intensive and time-consuming, but it may contribute to improving treatment strategies for this tumor, which is difficult to treat if local relapse occurs.

G. Ewing's Sarcoma

In Ewing's sarcoma, 90% of cases are characterized by the chromosomal translocation (11;22)(q24;q12). This rearrangement juxtaposes the 5′ portion from a newly described gene, termed EWS, to the 3′ part of the FLI-1 oncogene, which is thought to represent the genetic basis of Ewing's sarcoma. RNA transcripts from this fusion gene have been utilized successfully by several investigators to detect sarcoma cells in peripheral blood and bone marrow (60–63).

H. Lung Cancer

Several genes have been used to detect hematogenous dissemination of lung cancer, including cell-structure proteins

(64). The problem of nonspecific positive results has not yet been resolved convincingly. In one study involving 40 patients with advanced small cell lung cancer, 60% of blood samples and 60% of sputum samples tested positive for bombesin mRNA, which was not detected in healthy controls (Knebel-Doeberitz, personal communication). Mutated ras proto-oncogene and mutated p53 tumor-suppressor gene have also been used for detection of occult lung cancer cells in sputum and blood (65).

V. FUTURE PROSPECTS

The PCR detection of tumor cells can be a highly valuable and powerful tool. We are only just beginning to explore the reliability and clinical usefulness of this technology for the detection of minimal cancer. A rapidly increasing number of candidate genes are being identified for detection of a variety of tumors. In several instances, the presence of circulating tumor cells in the peripheral blood has proven to correlate with the extent of disease and to be of prognostic value. This technique could be helpful for studying tumor biology as well as for defining risk populations. This would be especially important for tumor types where adjuvant treatment strategies have been developed, since it may be possible to base treatment decisions on molecular staging in addition to conventional parameters.

It is, however, extremely important to develop this field with great caution. PCR is very sensitive to contamination. It has not been thoroughly investigated whether the rare illegitimate transcription of tumor-specific genes in normal cells may cause false positive results (66). Prior to widespread application, it is crucial to establish very rigid quality-assurance systems for academic centers as well as commercial laboratories. To establish clinical utility, large prospective studies are needed to test the prognostic value of PCR results

(10,11), since detection of occult tumor cells by PCR cannot automatically be viewed as a disease stage warranting systemic treatment.

REFERENCES

1. Osborne M, Wong GY. Asina S, Old LJ, Cote RJ, Rosen PP. Sensitivity on immunocytochemical detection of breast cancer cells in human bone marrow. Cancer Res 1991; 51:2706–2709.
2. Lindemann F, Schlimok G, Dirschedl P, Witte J, Riethmüller G. Prognostic significance of micrometastatic tumor cells in bone marrow of colorectal cancer patients. Lancet 1992; 340;685–689.
3. Cote RJ, Rosen PP, Lesser ML, Old LJ, Osborne MP. Prediction of early relapse in patients with operable breast cancer by detection of occult bone marrow micrometastases. J Clin Oncol 1991; 9:1749–1756.
4. Harbeck N, Untch M, Pache L, Eiermann W. Tumour cell detection in the bone marrow of breast cancer patients at primary therapy: Results of a 3 year median follow-up. Br J Cancer 1994; 69;566–571.
5. Manni JL, Easton D, Berger U, Gazet JC, Ford HT, Dearnhey D, Coombes RC. Bone marrow micrometastases in primary breast cancer: Prognostic significance after 6 years follow-up. Eur J Cancer 1991; 27:1552–1555.
6. Keilholz U (for the EORTC Melanoma Cooperative Group). Diagnostic PCR in Melanoma: Methods and Quality assurance. (Rev) Eur J Cancer, 1996; 32:1661–1663.
7. Chomczynski, P, Sacchi, N. Single step method of RNA isolation by acid guanidinium thiocynate-phenol-chloroform extraction. Anal Biochem 1987; 162:156.
8. Zaaijer HL, Cuypers HTM, Reesink HW, Winkel IN, Gerken G, Leslie PN. Reliability of polymerase chain reaction for detection of hepatitis C virus. Lancet 1993; 341:722–724.
9. Kwok S, Higuchi R. Avoiding false positives with PCR. Nature 1989, 339; 237–238.
10. Johnson PWM, Burchill SA, Selby PJ. The molecular detec-

tion of circulating tumour cells. (Rev) Br J Cancer 1995; 72;268–276.

11. Buzaid AC, Balch CM. Polymerase chain reaction of melanoma in peripheral blood: Too early to assess clinical value. J Natl Cancer Inst 1996; 88:569–570.

12. Adema G, de Boer AJ, van't Hullenaar R, Denijn M, Ruiter DJ, Vogel AM, Figdor CG. Melanocyte lineage-specific antigens recognized by monoclonal antibodies NKI-beteb, HMB-50, and HMB-45 are encoded by a single cDNA. Am J Path 1993; 143:1579–1585.

13. Adema GJ, de Boer AJ, Vogel AM, Loenen WA, Figdor CG. Molecular characterization of the melanoma linage specific antigen gp100. J Biol Chem 1994; 269:20126–20133.

14. Kawakami Y, Eliyahu S, Delgado CH, Robbins PF, Rivoltini L, Topalian SL, Miki T, Rosenberg SA. Cloning the gene coding for a shared human melanoma antigen recognized by autologous T cells infiltrating into tumor. Proc Natl Acad Sci USA 1994; 91:3515–3519.

15. Carrel S, Dore JF, Ruiter D, Prade M, Lejeune F, Kleeberg U, Rümke P, Bröcker E. The EORTC melanoma group exchange program: Evaluation of a multicenter monoclonal antibody study. Int J Cancer 1991; 48:836–847.

16. Scheibenbogen C, Weyers I, Ruiter D, Willhauck M, Bittinger A, Keilholz U. Expression of the melanocyte linage specific antigen gp100 in melanoma metastases prior to and following immunotherapy with IFNα and IL-2. Proceedings of ASCO 1996; 440.

17. Chen YT, Stockert E, Tsang S, Coplan KA, Old LJ. Immunophenotyping of melanomas for tyrosinase: Implications for vaccine development. Proc Natl Acad Sci USA 1995; 92:8125–8129.

18. Marincola FM, HiJazi YM, Fetsch P, Salgaller ML, Rivoltini L, Cormier J, Simonis TB, Duray PH, Herlyn M. Kawakami Y, Rosenberg SA. Analysis of expression of the melanoma-associated antigens MART-1 and gp100 in metastatic melanoma cell lines and in situ lesions. J Immunotherapy 1996; in press.

19. Coulie PG, V Brichard, A van Pel, T Wölfel, J Schneider, C Traversari, S Mattei, E de Plaen, C, Lurquin, JP Szikora, JC Renauld, T Boon. A new gene coding for a differentiation anti-

gen recognized by autologous cytoloytic T lymphocytes on HLA-A2 melanomas. J Exp Med 1994; 180:35–42.

20. Gaugler B, van den Eynde B, van der Bruggen P, et al. Human gene MAGE-3 codes for an antigen recognized on a melanoma by autologous cytoloytic T lymphocytes. J Exp Med 1994; 179:921–930.

21. Brasseur F, Rimoldi D, Lienard D, et al. Expression of MAGE genes in primary and metastatic cutaneous melanoma. Int J Cancer 1995; 63:375–380.

22. De Plaen E, Arden K, Traversari C, et al. Structure, chromosomal localization and expression of twelve genes of the MAGE family. Immunogenetics 1994; 40:360–369.

23. Smith B, Selby P, Southgate J, Pittman K, Bradley C, Blair GE. Detection of melanoma cells in peripheral blood by means of reverse transcriptase and polymerase chain reaction. Lancet 1991; 338:1227–1229.

24. Brossart P, Keilholz U, Willhauck M, Scheibenbogen C, Möhler T, Hunstein W. Hematogenous spread of malignant melanoma cells in different stages of disease. J Invest Dermatol 1993; 101:887–189.

25. Tobal K, Sherman LS, Foss AJ, Lightman SL. Detection of melanocytes from uveal melanoma in peripheral blood using the polymerase chain reaction. Invest Ophthalmol Vis Sci 1993; 34:2622–2625.

26. Brossart P, Keilholz U, Scheibenbogen C, Möhler T, Willhauck M, Hunstein W. Detection of residual tumor cells in patients with malignant melanoma responding to immunotherapy. J Immunother 1994; 15:38–41.

27. Battayani Z, Grob J, Xerri L, Noe C, Zarour H, Houvaeneghel G, Delpero JR, Birmbaum D, Hasssoun J, Bonerandi JJ. PCR detection of circulating melanocytes as a prognostic marker in patients with melanoma. Arch Dermatol 1995; 131:443–447.

28. Hoon DSB, Wang Y, Dale PS, Conrad AJ, Schmid P, Garrison D, Kuo C, Foshag LJ, Nizze AJ, Morton DL. Detection of occult melanoma cells in blood with a multiple-marker polymerase chain reaction assay. J Clin Oncol 1995; 13:2109–2116.

29. Foss AJ, Guille MJ, Occleston NL, Hykin PG, Hungerford JL, Lightman S. The detection of melanoma cells in peripheral

blood by reverse transcription-polymerase chain reaction. Br J Cancer 1995; 72:155–159.

30. Kunter U, Buer J, Probst M, Duensing S, Dallmann I, Gosse J, et al. Peripheral blood tyrosinase messanger RNA detection and survival in malignant melanoma. J Natl Cancer Inst 1996; 88:590–594.

31. Curry BJ, Smith MJ and Hersey P. Detection and quantitation of melanoma cells in the circulation of patients. Melanoma Res 1996; 6:45–54.

32. Brossart P, Schmier J, Krüger S, Willhauck M, Scheibenbogen C, Möhler T, Keilholz U. A PCR-based semiquantitative assessment of malignant melanoma cells in peripheral blood. Cancer Res 1995; 55:4065–4068.

33. Mellado B, Colomer D, Castel T, Munoz M, Galan M, Vives Corrons J, et al. Detection of circulating neoplastic cells by reverse-transcriptase polymerase chain reaction (RT-PCR) correlates with stage and prognosis in malignant melanoma. Proceedings of ASCO 1996; 433.

34. Wang X, Heller R, VanVoorhis N, Cruse CW, Glass F, Fenske N, Berman C, Leo-Messina J, Rappaport D, Wells K. Detection of submicroscopic lymph node metastases with polymerase chain reaction in patients with malignant melanoma. Ann Surg 1994; 220:768–774.

35. Moreno JG, Croce C,M, Fischer R, Monne M, Vikho P, Mulholland SG, Gomella L. Detection of hematogenous micrometastisis in patients with prostate cancer. Cancer Res 1992; 52:6110–6112.

36. Deguchi T, Doi T, Ehara H, Ito S, Takahashi Y, Nishino Y, Fujihiro S, Kawamura T, Komeda H, Horie M. Detection of micrometastatic prostate cancer cells in lymph nodes by reverse transcriptase polymerase chain reaction. Cancer Res 1993; 53:5350–5354.

37. Israeli RS, Miller WH, Su SL, Powell T, Fair WR, Samadi DS, Huryk RF, Deblasio A, Edwards ET, Wise GJ, Heston WDW. Sensitive nested reserve transcription polymerase chain reaction detection of circulating prostatic tumor cells: Comparison of prostate-specific membrane antigen and prostate-specific antigen-based assays. Cancer Res 1994; 54: 6306–6310.

38. Katz AE, Olsson CA, Raffo AJ, Cama C, Perlman H, Seaman E, O'Toole KM, McMahon D, Benson MC, Buttyan R. Molecular staging of prostate cancer with the use of an enhanced reverse transcriptase-PCR assay. Urology 1994; 43: 765–775.

39. Seiden MV, Kantoff PW, Krithivas K, Propert K, Bryant M, Haltom E, Gaynes L, Kaplan I, Bubley G, DeWolf W, et al. Detection of circulating tumor cells in men with localized prostate cancer. J Clin Oncol 1994; 12:2634–2639.

40. Ghossein RA, Scher HI, Gerald WL, Kelly WK, Curley T, Amsterdam A, Zhang ZF, Rosai J. Detection of circulating tumor cells in patients with localized and metastatic prostatic carcinoma: Clinical implications. J Clin Oncol 1995;13: 1195–1200.

41. Jaakkola S, Vornanen T, Leinonen J, Rannikko S, Stenman UH. Detection of prostatic cells in peripheral blood: Correlation with serum concentrations of prostate-specific antigen. Clin Chem 1995; 41:182–186.

42. Loric S, Dumas F, Eschwege P, Blanchet P, Benoit G, Jardin A, Lacour B. Enhanced detection of hematogenous circulating prostatic cells in patients with prostate adenocarcinoma by using nested reverse transcription polymerase chain reaction assay based on prostate-specific membrane antigen. Clin Chem 1995; 41:1698–1704.

43. Gerhard M, Juhl H, Kalthoff H, Schreiber HW, Wagener C, Neumaier M. Specific detection if carcinoembryonic antigen-expressing tumor cells in bone marrow aspirates by polymerase chain reaction. J Clin Oncol 1994; 12:725–729.

44. Sidransky D, Tokino T, Hamilton SR, Kinzler KW, Levin B, Frost P, Vogelstein B. Identification of ras oncogene mutations in the stool of patients with curable colorectal tumours. Science 1992; 256:102–105.

45. Almoguera C, Shibata D, Forrester K, Martin J, Arnheim H, Perucho M. Most human carcinomas of the exocrine pancreas contain mutant c-K-Ras genes. Cell 1988; 53:549–554.

46. Tada M, Omata M, Kawai S, Saisho H, Ohto M, Saiki RK, Sninsky JJ. Detection of ras gene mutations in pancreatic juice and peripheral blood of patients with pancreatic adenocarcinoma. Cancer Res 1993; 53:2472–2474.

47. Burchill SA, Bradbury MF, Pittman K, Southgate J, Smith B, Selby P. Detection of epithelial cancer cells in peripheral blood by reverse transcriptase polymerase chain reaction. Br J Cancer 1994c; 71:278–281.

48. Neumaier M, Gerhard M, Wagener C. Diagnosis of micrometastases by the amplification of tissue-specific genes. Gene 1995; 159:43–47.

49. Datta YH, Adams PT, Drobyski WR, Ethier SP, Terry VH, Roth MS. Sensitive detection of occult breast cancer by the reverse transcriptase polymerase chain reaction. J. Clin. Oncol 1994; 12:475–482.

50. Matsumura Y, Tarin D. Significance of CD44 gene products for cancer diagnosis and disease evaluation. Lancet 1992; 340:1053–1058.

51. Krismann M, Todt B, Schroder J, Gareis D, Muller KM, Seeber S, Schutte J. Low specificity of cytokeratin 19 reverse transcriptase-polymerase chain reaction analyses for detection of hematogenous lung cancer dissemination. J Clin Oncol 1995; 13:2769–2775.

52. Schoenfeld A, Luqmani E, Smith D, Oreilly S, Shousha S, Sinnet HD, Coombes RC. Detection of breast cancer micrometastases in axillary lymph-nodes by using poylmerase chain reaction. Cancer Res 1994; 54:2986–2990.

53. Brown DC, Purushotham AD, Birnie GD, George WD. Detection of intraoperative tumor cell dissemination in patients with breast cancer by use of reverse transcription and polymerase chain reaction. Surgery 1995; 117:95–101.

54. Naito H, Kuzumaki N, Uchino J-I, Kobayashi R, Shikano T, Ishikawa Y, Matsumoto S. Detection of tyrosine hydroxylase mRNA and minimal neuroblastoma cells by the reverse transcription—polymerase chain reaction. Eur j Cancer 1991; 27:762–765.

55. Mattano LA, Moss TJ, Emerson SG. Sensitive detection of rare circulating neuroblastoma cells by the reverse transcriptase-polymerase chain reaction. Cancer Res 1992; 52: 4701–4705.

56. Burchill SA, Bradbury FM, Smith B, Lewis IJ, Selby P. Neuroblastoma cell detection by reverse transcriptase polymerase

chain reaction (rt-PCR) for tyrosine hydroxylase messenger RNA. Int J Cancer 1994a; 57:671–675.

57. Miyajima Y, Kato K, Numata S, Kudo K, Horibe K. Detection of neuroblastoma cells in bone marrow and peripheral blood at diagnosis by the reverse transcriptase-polymerase chain reaction for tyrosine hydroxylase mRNA. Cancer 1995; 75:2757–2761.

58. Butturini A, Chen RL, Tang SQ, Hong CM, Peters J, Matthay KK, et al. Detection of bone marrow (BM) metastases in neuroblastoma (NBL) by RT-PCR for neural and tumor associated genes. Proceedings of ASCO 1996; 468.

59. Brennan JA, Mao L, Hruban RH, Boyle JO, Eby YJ, Koch WM, et al. Molecular assessment of histopathological staging in squamous cell carcinoma of the head and neck. N Engl J Med 1995; 332:429–435.

60. Pfleiderer C, Zoubek A, Gruber B, Kronberger M, Ambros PF, Lion T, Fink FM, Gadner H, Kovar H. Detection of tumour cells in peripheral blood and bone marrow from Ewing tumour patients by RT-PCR. Int J Cancer 1995; 64:135–139.

61. Delattre O, Zucman J, Melot T, Garau XS, Zucker JM, Lenoir GM, Ambros PF, Sheer D, Turccarel C, Triche TJ. The Ewing family of tumors—a subgroup of small round cell tumors defined by specific chimeric transcripts. N Engl J Med 1994; 331:294–299.

62. Peter M, Magdelenat H, Michon J, Melot T, Oberlin O, Zucker JM, Thomas G, Delattre O. Sensitive detection of occult Ewing's cells by the reverse transcriptase-polymerase chain reaction. Br J Cancer 1995; 72:96–100.

63. Zoubek A, Pfleiderer C, Ambros PF, Kronberger M, Dworzak MN, Gruber B, Luegmayer A, Windhager R, Fink FM, Urban C, et al. Minimal metastatic and minimal residual disease in patients with Ewing tumours. Klin Padiatr 1995; 207: 242–247.

64. Krismann M, Todt B, Gareis D, Müller KM, Seeber S, Schütte J. Low specifity of cytokeratin 19 reverse transcriptase-polymerase chain reaction analyses for detection of hematogenous lung cancer detection. J Clin Oncol 1995; 13: 2769–2775.

65. Mao L, Hruban RH, Boyle JO, Tockmann M, Sidransky D. Detection of oncogene mutations in sputum precedes the diagnosis of lung cancer. Cancer Res 1994; 54:1634–1637.

66. Chelly J, Concordet JP, Kaplan JC, Kahn A: Illegitimate transcription: Transcription of any gene in any cell. Proc Natl Acad Sci USA 1989; 86:2617–2621.

INDEX

ABOUT THE EDITOR

JOHN M. KIRKWOOD is Director of the Melanoma Center at the University of Pittsburgh Cancer Institute and Professor and Vice Chairman for Clinical Research in the Department of Medicine at the University of Pittsburgh School of Medicine, Pittsburgh, Pennsylvania. The author or coauthor of over 160 professional papers, book chapters, and reviews, and over 190 abstracts that reflect his research interests in the diagnosis, course, and treatment of melanoma, he is a member of the American Federation for Clinical Research, the American Society for Clinical Oncology, the American Association for Cancer Research, the National Cancer Foundation, the Society for Biologic Therapy, and the International Society for Interferon Research, among other organizations, and serves on the editorial boards of multiple journals. Dr. Kirkwood has chaired the Biologics Committee of the Eastern Cooperative Oncology Group (ECOG) and currently is chairman of the ECOG's Melanoma Committee. He received the A.B. degree (1969) in biochemistry from Oberlin College, Ohio, and the M.D. degree (1973) from Yale University School of Medicine, New Haven, Connecticut. Dr. Kirkwood is certified by the American Board of Internal Medicine in Medical Oncology.